Menopause Can Be Fun

Written and illustrated by
Allene G. Hatch

ISBN-13: 978-1456371180

ISBN-10: 1456371185

MENOPAUSE CAN BE FUN

Marriage is the price men pay for sex; sex is the price women pay for marriage.

— *Anonymous*

ACKNOWLEDGMENT

I wish to express my eternal gratitude to Harlan D. Root, M.D. for carefully checking and editing my 1973 book to see that all the medical facts therein were still viable in the present day. The main change in medical procedure is that rarely and selectively is estrogen therapy recommended by any gynecologist. Too many lethal side effects such as strokes, heart attacks, and cervical and breast cancer were discovered in the past thirty seven years. That chance, plus the arrival of Viagra on the scene are the two main differences between then, 1973 and now, 20010.

Otherwise, Dr. Root said that the facts about menopause contained in the book are still viable and should be very reassuring and helpful to all women (and men) who are coping with the vicissitudes of this unsettling period in their lives. Dr. Root is emphatic about this and I thank him once again for encouraging me to republish my book for exactly that purpose.

AUTHOR'S NOTE

The additions and amendments in this text, which was originally published in the 1970s, are indicated by the use of French {or "curly"} brackets, to distinguish them from parenthetical phrases that occurred in the original.

CHAPTER ONE

All women's problems start with MEN. Not just men themselves, but their spoor, their tracks bedevil the English language.

Think of the pivotal words in a woman's life; her sexual problems start with the Menarche, meaning the beginning of *men*struation and supposedly cease with *men*opause. In between we have *men*acing, *men*dacious *man* making us *men*dicants. We become *men*ials with *men*tal problems. Moving into the singular, it becomes *man*ifest that we are *man*euvered, *man*aged, *man*gled even *man*ducated by *man*gy, *man*ner-less, *man*iacal *man* himself. When faced with these irrefutable facts, a man will fix you with a steely eye and mutter, "Bull *man*ure." Unless, of course, he has heard of the Anglo-Saxon equivalent. If so, he will use it.

There are 135 words beginning with 'men' and 393 words beginning with 'man' in Webster's Unabridged Dictionary; the grand total being 528. Add seven words beginning with 'male' and you have 535.

However, the word female is listed only twice and has a mere 19 derivations. Lump them in with the 17 listings for woman words and you get a big 36. How can people possibly doubt that we were made from Adam's rib! Had the Lord used the lower mandible we could have been called the jawbone of an ass, which would carry out the stubborn logic of man calling us woman — a man plus a womb, and/or female — a male plus a fetus.

But we must assume that God wasn't facetious when he created us. As women — females — we are much too serious-minded to like being a perpetual joke, albeit some of us are. No, *He* was earnest but *He* didn't have a good panel of advisors. (No women.) Also, *He* was on very safe ground. *He* would never have to live with one of us, never have to roar for clean socks and never, never have to survive the companionship of a wife who was going through menopause at the same time his teenage youngsters were rocking and rolling through puberty. Good staff work, that.

He left it for man to suffer woman to come unto him, for man to try to perfect us imperfect creatures in his own image—to tell us how to behave, what to think, what to wear, even tell us what subjects are proper to discuss. Menopause apparently isn't one of them for although feminism is rampant in this latter part of the 20th Century, and books about sexual deviations of any and all kinds are hitting the bestseller lists, the phases of menopause are, unlike the moon, still shrouded in myth and mystery. Man has put it on the "no-no" list.

Your friendly gynecologist murmurs blandly, "You're just fine; nothing to worry about." And if asked a delicate question, your friendly family clergyman will either faint or run away. Husbands are notoriously unsympathetic about what they term female frailties, so instead of being soothed and cosseted, which surely is our due, we are told to buck up, stop being neurotic, take a Milltown, take a trip, keep busy, etc., etc.

Of course, the whole problem started back with Adam's missing rib. Once Eve had two good feet under her and a mind of her own, she cozied up to the snake and ate the apple. That did it. Fig leaves, disillusionment and the curse. A mean price to pay for the chance of a torrid sex life. The greatest malediction was, of course, the creation of woman's desire for man.

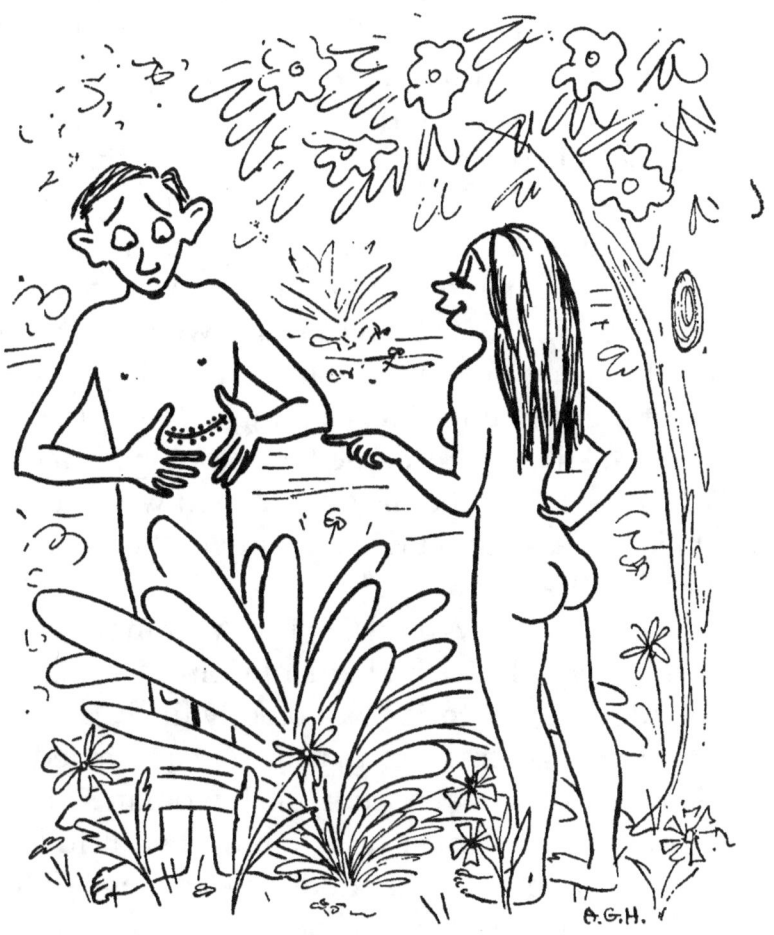

Man immediately decided that the subject of woman's monthly period was taboo. She was hustled to a secluded place to spend her "unclean" time alone and in disgrace. Her involuntary solitude was called many things by many peoples through the ages, and "Ishnati" by our own not-so-sweet Sioux.

Man became so obsessed with making woman realize this humiliation that the subject of blood when applied to women was unmentionable. In the 16th Century Johnnie Armstrong said with true Scottish insouciance, "I'll lay me dune and bleed awhile and then rise up and fight again." Joan of Arc could never have gotten away with a crack like that. Or take Lady Macbeth muttering in horror, "I never knew the old man had so much blood in him." Any family doctor faced with a hemorrhaging female would be tarred and feathered if he expressed a like opinion.

The Victorians made "bloody" into a swear word in the 19th century. In the 20th Century we have Teddy Roosevelt, always prone to bashing himself up in the pursuit of the strenuous life, arriving at the front door of Sagamore Hill, a crimson tide enveloping his face.

"Teddy dear," sighed his exasperated wife, "if you must bleed, please don't do so on my best carpets; go and bleed in the bathroom."

Reverse the sexes. Would George Washington have said that to Martha? Abraham Lincoln to Mrs. Lincoln, or Albert to Victoria? Not bloody likely.

Man, thorough creature that he is, has carried his obsession to its logical conclusion. If woman's blood-letting propensities must be ignored, then it follows that the stopping of her habitual flow (change of life) must also be ignored. So, although everything else about the human female—her face, her figure, her foibles, her psyche, her prowess in the kitchen, in the office, in the arts, in bed, in the nude, and in the news, has become a happy hunting ground for writers from Kinsey to Kerouac and no nugget of information is too small to escape exhaustive examination and explanation, menopause has not yet become grist for the

4

male mill. They are scared witless of the subject. Since we've been brainwashed for centuries by the dominant sex, so are we.

A dancer with seven veils is no more elusive than the knotty subject before us; the alteration of our own bodies. Let's give a tug at the first veil.

The outer layer, an amorphous smoky one, conceals the entire shape of the form beneath. Impenetrable at first glance, we soon perceive it is the mist of inaccessibility. The knowledge we don't have or the half-truths we do, shifts in each breeze of speculation.

I remember as a child having only heard hushed whispers in corners about the subject, I became convinced there was something grown-ups did, rather scary (else why the whispers?), called "meadowpause"! We lived on a farm and cows grazing peacefully in the fields were an everyday sight. I wondered if Mummy was going out to eat grass with the cows and linger awhile. Grown-ups did so many silly things anyhow.

Having been guilty of eavesdropping, I was somewhat shy about asking Mummy to explain the word. But at six my bump of curiosity was fully developed, so I finally asked her when she was going out and meadowpause?"

As she looked slightly startled, I quickly added that I wanted to go along too.

"What do you think 'meadowpause' means?" from Mummy.

"Just what it says," from literal me. "You go out and stand in the meadow very quietly with the cows."

"Well, being put out to pasture is as good a definition as I've heard yet," was my mother's reply.

"Let's let it go at that. Don't worry, I won't go out and 'meadowpause' for awhile yet."

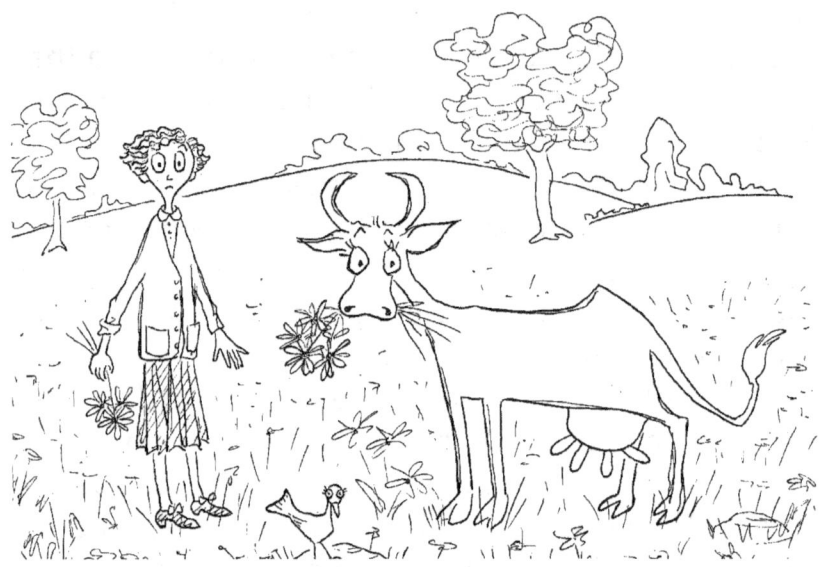

Actually, that was the only discussion my mother and I ever had about sex. Eleven years later when mummy was in the hospital recovering from a hysterectomy, I was still so vague about the feminine interior that I happily presented her with two books I knew she'd love. One was a new anthology called *The Book of the Opera* and the other was my beloved James Thurber's latest treatise entitled *Is Sex Necessary?*

Not wishing to hurt my feelings, Mummy thanked me politely at the time.

Therefore, I was surprised during my next visit to find myself in the doghouse.

"I don't know why you brought me that Thurber book; I've had nurses in here all day long for days."

"But it's a great book, Mummy, very funny. Have you read it?"

"I haven't had a chance. The nurses don't know

who Thurber is. They think it's a medical book and they keep coming to find out if sex really is necessary."

To complete the picture of my post-Victorian ignorance, I remember thinking at about the same time, having just started necking with boys, what a bore marriage must be, since then you could kiss your husband any time you wanted to, thus taking all the excitement out of it. I hasten to add that my older sister had informed me how and where babies came from, but I assumed sexual intercourse was rather like brushing one's teeth and one performed the onerous task only when one wished to start a family.

Saint Paul and I would have gotten along just fine.

The same veil of hushed whispers about menopause that existed in the 1930s exists today. I have yet to have a friend say to me "Played a great game of golf yesterday. Went around in 89 with only three hot flashes."

No, they either get a deep tan or use makeup the color of a Native American because the man-instilled feeling of disgrace makes them hide any symptoms they possibly can.

That is why I think the time has come to take the bull by the horns (no castrating female, I) and have a good look at the forbidden subject — Menopause.

CHAPTER TWO

Webster's Dictionary says tersely:

menopause, m. (*Meno* and Gr. *pausis*, a cessation). The period of natural cessation of menstruation; change of life.

The first definition is put quite poetically for a dictionary — cessation of menstruation — it is the phrase "change of life" that strikes terror to the heart. Forty-odd years of getting accustomed to living on this planet, living with family and friends; twenty-odd years of adjusting to a job and/or husband and children, then *whammo*, everything we've learned so painfully is about to be turned topsy-turvy by a man-invented phrase: change of life. Suddenly we're being swept towards the edge of Niagara Falls with no hope of rescue in sight. Our life is about to be altered and everyone has clammed up.

Having destroyed the veil of inaccessibility, or rather taboo, let's tackle the next filmy deceiver; that scary phrase, that shibboleth, "change of life," surely as diabolical and insidious a collection of words as man ever dreamed up to confound and confuse woman. It implies that we haven't been having a "change of life" ever since we were born.

The most traumatic change in our lives comes when we are pushed helpless and screaming into the world from a nice, safe, warm womb. Man in his infinite wisdom gave that somewhat messy procedure the poetic name of birth. Awe, mystery, worship, romance have always surrounded the fact of birth. At least one great religion is based on a virgin variation thereof. There weren't enough good words in any language to praise

9

birth per se until Margaret Sanger came along with her revolutionary plans for controlling a too fecund population.

Once down-to-earth Mrs. Sanger had made birth control a public issue the knotty problem of birth control entered the political arena along with thousands of dedicated women. That was certainly a historic change of life for a female of any age.

Returning to our individual lives, after our natal day we start what is to be a continual series of changes; some gradual, as our everyday growth; and some rather rude changes, like puberty. We change schools, ideas, ideals, politics, clothes, hairdos, even friends, like so many feckless chameleons. Every cell in the body is said to be replaced every seven years. And the majority of us long for the greatest change of all in our lives, i.e., enticing some very wary male into a state of wedded bliss. Having accomplished that, we await even more eagerly further changes called children. We do all this with endless enthusiasm and gusto so we shouldn't boggle at one-more change in our forties. Man is not the only one who can be master of his fate and captain of his soul; lashed to the mast and a little sea-sick, we can still navigate. After all, most figureheads on the old sailing ships were buxom ladies, hence the phrase "breasting the waves."

A good example of feminine intrepidity to mull over on a rainy day is the flamboyant, piratical Irish Queen, Gracia O'Malley, who reigned in the time of Good Queen Bess. On her way to pay her respects to Queen Elizabeth I, she was delivered of a son while a fearful storm made truth of the phrase "high seas." When Gracia arrived at court, her august rival offered

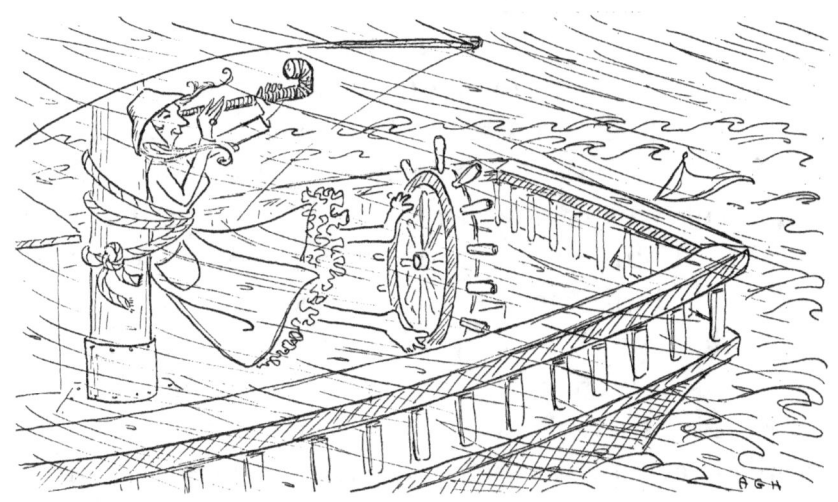

to give the newborn lad an English title. Queen Gracia answered tartly that her son would become a King of Ireland, enough title for anyone, thank you. She returned to Ireland with her head intact and continued her predatory ways. Not just at sea either. On land she was wont to marry some poor soul for a coveted castle. Once she had his domain firmly in her grasp, she then booted him out in his last suit of armor: not a queen for all seasons.

I don't offer Gracia O'Malley's manners as an object of emulation, just her fortitude. Queen baiting and piracy not being exactly a current form of relaxation for most of us, let us concentrate on where the guts come from to pursue such bizarre activities. I would say from pride, courage and self-knowledge, sometimes known as moxie. With these characteristics we can face anything, the high seas, a condescending queen — or menopause.

So if we analyze this second veil, that of fear, born of the ominous slogan "change of life" with a little effort we can see it for what it is: a psychological bugbear. Out damned spot. We are only afraid of the unknown or as President Roosevelt once said so aptly to our depression-ridden country, "You have nothing to fear but fear itself." We have been trained to take pride in ourselves, we are now armed with courage, therefore let us gird our loins with physical self-knowledge.

We are built the way we are because we women were designed as baby-making machines. Let the feminists howl to the stars, that's the ball-game, girls. Our entire system swings to the rhythm of the hormone beat. (Hormones obviously control the male body, too, but we will come to that later.) In our case the endocrine system involves the liver, the pituitary, thyroid, parathyroid, and adrenal glands plus the ovaries. Our bodily functions are controlled by these tiny powerhouses; the adrenals produce 45 different hormones for instance. But our interest is in the part of the endocrine system that controls our sexuality — the pituitary and adrenal glands and the ovaries.

The pituitary gland controls all bodily functions and thus is known as the master gland. In the menstrual cycle it is the coach who calls the signals. The pituitary produces the FSH (follicle stimulating hormone) which at puberty starts the development of the ovaries and once started periodically sends FSH through the bloodstream to get the ovaries cracking. When hit with a blast of FSH a cluster of follicles (hair-like objects on the surface of the ovaries) starts to swell. Usually only one of the budding group becomes an egg, the follicle of which then starts sending extra quantities of estrogen to the uterus to start jazzing up the would-be nursery. Estrogen thickens up

12

its walls, stores away little goodies for the hoped-for arrival to munch on and generally makes itself very useful, like rolling out the red carpet down the vagina for the expected sperm by making the chemistry simpatico {and causes breast engorgement.}

About two weeks after the original signal the pituitary gland sends out a shot of LH (luteinizing hormone.) At this signal the ripened egg bursts from its follicle and is grabbed by the waving tentacles of the Fallopian tube to start its three-day journey to the uterus. The minute the egg leaves the follicle the ruptured sac known as the corpus luteum begins to pour out the secondary ovarian hormone—progesterone. It not only calms down the other excited follicles but rushes off to the uterus to help the overworked estrogen decorate the nursery. More lining for the walls, more food and a definite slowing down of the rhythmic contractions of the womb so that the ovum will be able to settle in comfortably, God willing and if the creeks don't rise. In case of pregnancy it also is ready to tell the breasts to start the milk production machinery going.

The egg spends another three days hanging around the womb hopefully waiting to be fertilized. If nothing happens its doom is sealed. The build-up of excess progesterone in the system flashes a signal to the pituitary which in turn cuts off its supply of LH to the empty follicle which in turn stops making progesterone and withers away. Like a stack of cards falling as soon as the soothing effects of progesterone on the uterine muscles ceases all hell breaks loose. The would-be nursery walls start expanding and contracting, smashing up the furniture, the vintage bottles of

13

blood — the works, and a general housecleaning takes place. Everything out! The poor scorned unfertilized egg is rushed through the general melée, unnoticed and unmourned. *Tant pis.* Another menstrual cycle has come and gone and another is on its way.

The fascinating thing about the two sets of hormones, the ones from the pituitary gland and the local ones from the ovaries, is their oscillating interaction. That's what keeps the ball game going, like the old song says: "You can't have one without the other."

The Textbook of Medical Physiology admits to science's limited understanding of the problem when it says blandly, "For reasons not understood, the adenohypophysis (pituitary gland) secretes a greatly enhanced amount of LH (Luteinizing Hormone) on the day immediately before ovulation. It has been postulated that at this time in the sexual cycle estrogen and progesterone exert a positive feedback effect on the secretion of LH rather than the normal negative feedback. This supposedly results from altered sensitivity of the hypothalamus to the estrogen and progesterone ... the cause of this effect is not known."

Any woman who has had her usual cranky, weepy pre-ovulation blues could tell them: it's the moon, boys, it's the moon!

Where we begin to run into real trouble as females, usually sometime between the ages of 45 and 50 (every medical book seems to have different magical ages) is when the shop starts to close down and the hormones stop playing their game of "one-o-cat" and go home.

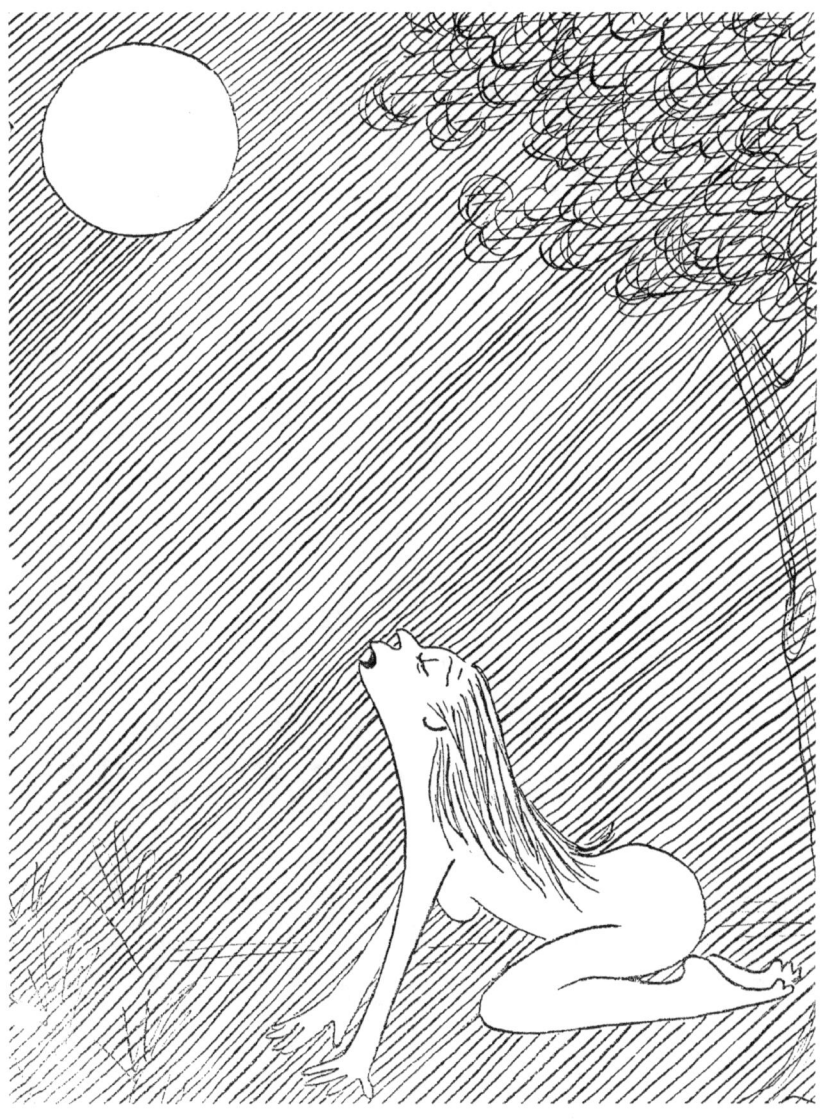

CHAPTER THREE

One of the lovely effects of our hormonal activity is our femininity: soft skin, firm flesh, shiny hair, musical voices, round hips that give us a distinctive way of walking and last, but hardly least, those twin orbs extolled by poets — our breasts. We were created toothsome and attractive to beguile the opposite sex so all our glorious baby-making paraphernalia wouldn't stand idle.

One ingenious anthropologist has come up with the theory (be prepared for a shift from the Bible to Darwin) that originally when our ancestors were scampering around on all fours, furry and fast, the most alluring part of a female's anatomy was the smooth, hairless posterior, winking and shimmering as she nimbly eluded her pursuer. Nicely placed for a quick grab by an alert male, and sensibly placed for a female, since, when bored she had only to sit down quickly to cover up her sex appeal.

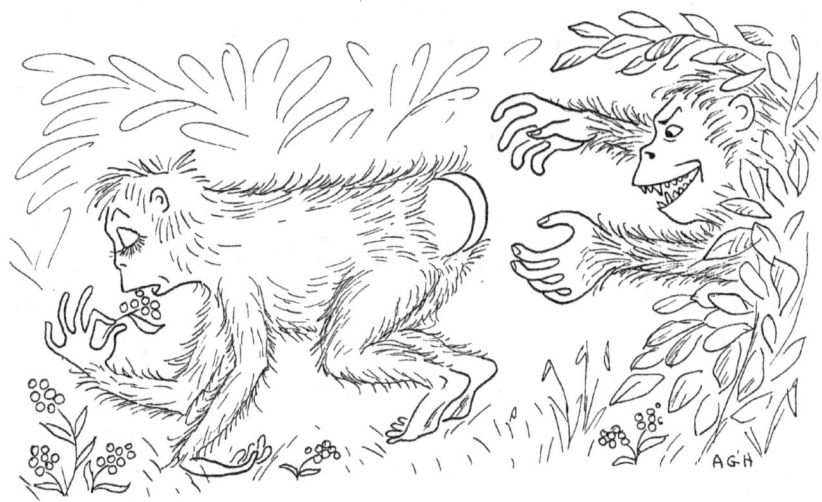

However, ape man soon started his upward climb to civilization, first by grabbing a stick and then by standing on his two hind legs, the better to swing it. The female, not to be outdone, stood up too, thus gaining dignity but losing her greatest asset. Nature, undeterred in her inexorable quest for more play-toys in the evolutionary game, took what had been female's rudimentary paps, designed for the easy feeding of the young, and enlarged them. Voilà! Breasts had made the scene. They joggled and bobbled even more

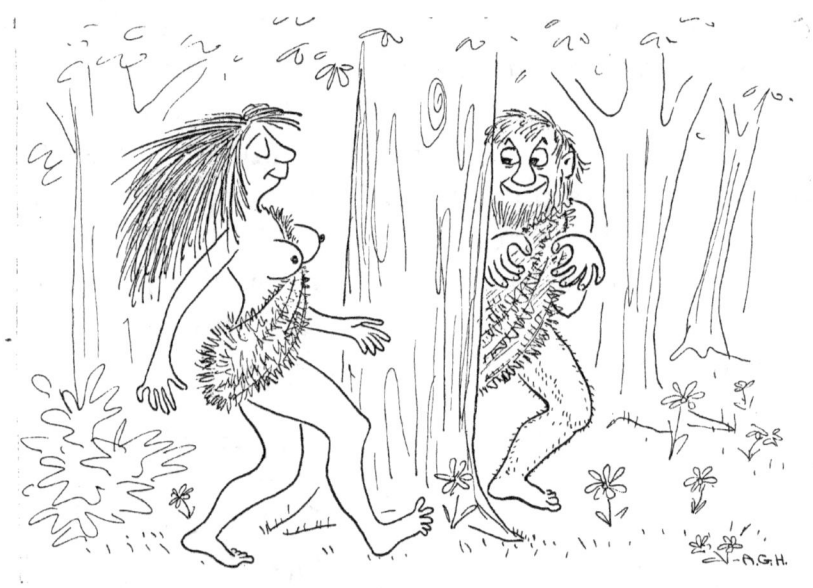

enticingly than buttocks, with the added convenience of being grab-able from all angles. No longer could a female sit down and feel safe. However, we still have atavistic types in our midst who prefer the posterior, known as tail-men. The Italian male has made fanny appreciation a high art-science, as anyone who has been pinched in the streets of Rome can attest. One tweak is worth a thousand words.

18

The thought of losing all these hard-won and highly developed feminine attributes in the course of menopause is a very depressing one. Luckily doctors and research scientists have cleverly devised ways of preserving them in spite of the fact that, whether we are a whim from Adam's rib or descended from a long line of hairy apes, there finally comes a period to our periods.

Every medical book, as I mentioned before, gives a different normal age for the "climacteric," as they choose to call menopause. It's nice to know that we females still baffle the medical profession. Some say 44 to 48, others 45 to 50, still others 45 to 55. Women have been known to bear children at 60, and some have experienced change of life in their 30s or even 20s. It all depends on our individual inner clock, so like good girl scouts we should be prepared any time from our early 40s on.

The Textbook of Medical Physiology provides this terse bloodless description:

"The term 'female climacteric' means the entire time, lasting from several months to several years during which the sexual cycles become irregular and gradually stop. In this period the woman must readjust her life from one that has been physiologically stimulated by estrogen production to one devoid of this feminizing hormone. The secretion of estrogen decreases rapidly and essentially no progesterone is secreted after the last ovulatory cycle. The loss of the estrogen often causes marked physiologic changes in the function of the body, including:

1. 'hot flashes' characterized by extreme flushing of the skin,

2. psychic sensations of dyspnea (difficulty breathing),
3. irritability
4. fatigue,
5. anxiety
6. depression
7. occasionally various psychotic states."

When I read this list to my husband, he said, "My God, you've been having change of life for the last twenty years!"

Menopause occurs in the female when the ovaries apparently "burn out." Our original supply of folli-cles in the ovaries is limited (the more you have, the later your menopause); when they are used up the hormonal rhythm is broken. No more follicles to be stimulated by the pituitary hormones into making ova, so the production of estrogen decreases in a cut-back reaction and gradually ceases altogether. And no more corpus luteans, so no more progesterone. However the adrenal gland continues to produce a small quantity of estrogen, more in some women than in others. {Some androgen is produced also.}

Since, as Dr. Robert B. Greenblatt says in Search the Scriptures, "the higher centers of the brain tem-per the activity of the pituitary glands, and the endo-crines respond to the nervous system," we find that our changing interior can be bolloxed up even more by our brain; i.e. worry can cause psychosomatic dis-turbances. Under stress the neurotic becomes more so. Also, when the ovaries stop producing estrogen, the pituitary responds by producing more gonadotro-pin hormones.

It is this increasing imbalance in our inner chemistry that is responsible for the previously mentioned list of symptoms. The loss of estrogen can also tend to let extra fat settle around the hips unless one is very active physically. While all this mayhem is taking place inside, sometimes extra amounts of testosterone (yes, Virginia, we do have a bit of that male hormone in our bodies) are produced and certain unpleasant things can result. Since testosterone stimulates the sebaceous glands of the skin to pour out more oil, acne can appear, plus unwanted facial hair. Testosterone also seems to be a sneaky aphrodisiac for the unsuspecting female.

Knowing all this we can see why estrogen becomes all-important around this time and why more and more doctors {used to} prescribe estrogen pills to return our body to normal behavior. {Recently it has been discovered that estrogen administration may increase the possibility of developing breast and uterine cancers. Thus, prescribing estrogen to control the symptoms of menopause has been markedly reduced.} But never take any hormone pills without a prescription from your gynecologist. Cysts or tumors can result from a sudden imbalance in the hormone level if you have a tendency that way. One reason why doctors feel that the longer, gradual menopause poses fewer problems is that it gives the system plenty of time to adjust.

I have a sneaking suspicion that the French have always had some secret weapon in that direction. I think it was Christian Dior who said he much preferred designing dresses for women over forty because only then did females begin to have style and really become attractive. The freedom a woman feels to develop her own personality, once released from child-bearing and rearing responsibilities, undoubtedly has something to do with this.

Then there is Rudyard Kipling's wonderful poem, "My Rival," about the gauche seventeen-year old girl always put in the shade by a fascinating, sophisticated beauty of forty-nine, which ends with the upbeat:

But even She must older grow
And end Her dancing days.
She can't go forever so
At concerts, balls and plays.
One ray of priceless hope I see
Before my footsteps shine:
Just think, that She'll be eighty-one
When I am forty-nine!

The greatest example of the durability of feminine beauty and charm must always be Ninon de Lenclos, a lively lady at Louis XIV's court, who kept a series of much younger lovers completely captivated and ardent until she was eighty. Her wit and sense made Larochefoucauld consult her about his maxims, Moliere about his comedies, and Scarron about his romances. When she was 56, her son, age 19, not knowing of their relationship, fell madly in love with her. When Ninon told the boy that she was his mother, he blew his brains out in a fit of pique. All of this devastation without hormones or vitamins.

Ninon's friend, Madame de Maintenon, as virtuously uptight as Ninon was swingingly loose, was the only woman to refuse to become Louis XIV's mistress. She was forty at the time. But eight long, proper years later, after the Queen's death, Madame de Maintenon consented to become the Sun King's secret morganatic wife, virtue being more than its own reward.

If we need added proof that our fifth decade is a great place to be, think of Elizabeth Barrett who bowled over Robert Browning when she was in her fortieth year. Theirs was such a wildly romantic love affair that Browning penned "take away love and our earth is a tomb."

In the past century we have beautiful, Junoesque 43-year-old Mrs. Galt walking out of the elevator on the second floor of the White House and into the arms of President Woodrow Wilson. It was love at first bump for both of them, although Mrs. Wilson admitted to me with great satisfaction, "I did notice that the President had on a tacky old suit, while I was wearing a beautifully cut black wool dress from Worths with a bunch of violets at my throat." She remained beautiful and feminine in her eighties as did the famous Colette who said longingly on her eightieth birthday, "If only one were 58, because at that time one is still desired and full of hope for the future."

"I cite these few cases to reassure any worried readers that their charm for — or interest in — or enjoyment of the opposite sex will not suddenly cease after menopause. Far from it: all the medical books agree that the average woman feels much better physically after the change and enjoys her sex life even more than before. Years of worry about unwanted pregnancies are suddenly removed from the marital bed or any other bed that you might happen to occupy.

Things look better already.

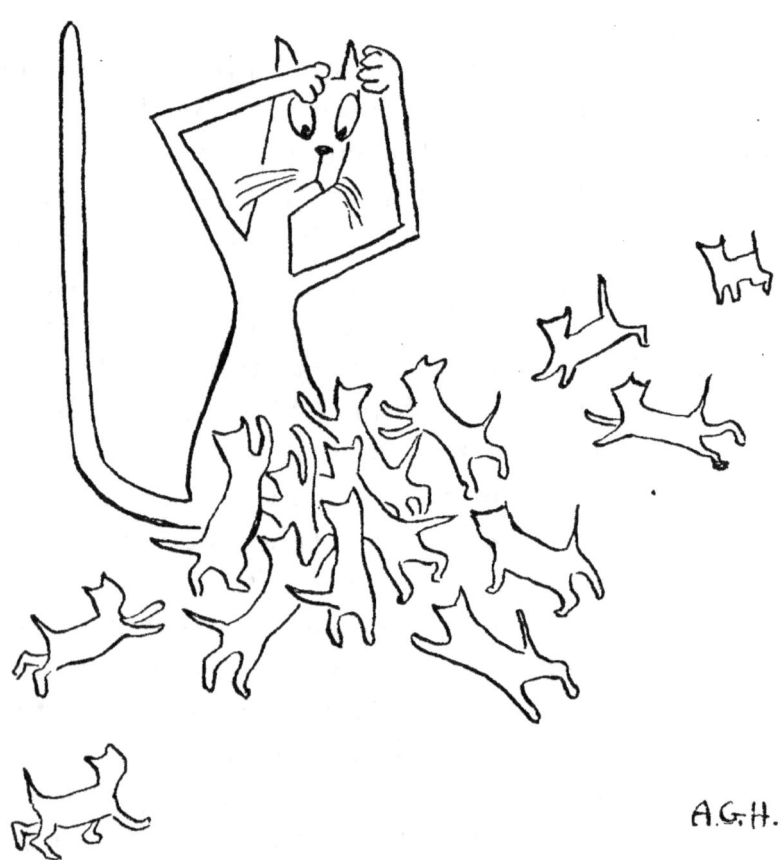

A.G.H.

CHAPTER FOUR

Let's become a combination of Pollyanna and Candide for a bit and think of how lucky we women are in "this best of all possible worlds."

Imagine if our reproductive organs had been designed similar to those of a chicken. One minute scratching happily around the barnyard, the next minute *"Wham, bam, thank you ma'am,"* attacked from the rear by a fresh rooster — and we wind up on the next. Naturally, laying a much larger egg (crunch!) and sitting and brooding a hell of a lot longer — nine months. What a big fat bore that would be. We may feel put upon chained to one of those House Beautiful's beautiful houses, but how much worse to be glued to a moldy, smelly pile of straw.

If we were fish, we wouldn't even have a feathery salute in passing. Having laid our eggs in some quiet backwater, we would swim away. A strange male fish would then wander by and "spread the sperm." As it was so neatly put in *Auntie Mame*: "Dull, duller, dullest." No wonder fish look so glassy-eyed.

Cats and dogs have a more interesting sex life, but unfortunately the more interesting it is, the busier the poor female becomes — bearing, raising and training litter after litter. No time left for a quick martini or a game of bridge; just *pant, pant, pant.* When you get to elephants, it's whoopee once a year whether you like it or not. When the male elephant is in "must," he must. Females either say yes or run like hell.

No other animal besides homo sapiens has arranged his sex life so satisfactorily, with or without the help of Sigmund Freud and Masters and Johnson.

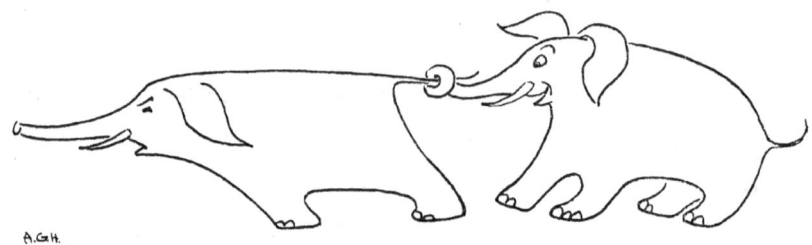

A.G.H.

Psychiatrist James A. Brussel says most soothingly, "Sex is an instinct and an instinct never dies."

So first of all we must count our blessings, such as they are, and then concentrate on solving our problems...what there are of them.

The second most soothing thing to learn about the mean-old-pause (the first being that our sex life won't come to a stumbling stop, is that eighty percent of all females never have any disagreeable symptoms at all. Apparently the less trouble you expect, the less you get, as in most situations. The menstrual periods remain normal but gradually become spaced further apart, the flow lessening, the periods finally stopping. {Sometimes the periods are erratic with spotting in between.} This takes from a year to eighteen months in most cases. A few sports take longer.

The next most fortunate group of women have only a few minor symptoms, easily taken care of with simple medication. In the case of restlessness and insomnia, doctors usually prescribe a mild sedative with a double dose at bedtime to ensure sleep.

I have long been an occasional user of sleeping pills when I am tense of overtired and can't get to sleep, and of tranquilizers when I find myself in an overemotional state. I am now a regular taker of estrogen pills as I begin to find myself waking up in the morning furious with everything — the world, myself and especially my poor, innocent husband.

Trying to stem my wrathful tirades, Alden might say, quite logically, "Why do you always blame me for everything?" to which I would reply with equal logic, "Because you're the only one around, that's why!"

When I told my gynecologist about my morning nasties he suggested a light dosage of estrogen to calm me down with a double dose the week before my period if needed, as that is when a female's own supply of estrogen is at its lowest ebb. Doctors say that lack of estrogen can cause aggressive behavior and in my case it is unfortunately true. {It would not be prescribed today.}

The menopause is a good time to begin thinking about vitamins and diet if you haven't before; the idea being that the healthier one is, the less wear and tear there is on the system. Dr. Joyce Brothers also points out in her book Woman that sufficient rest becomes extremely important during the climacteric. She says "Adolescents, pregnant women and women experiencing menopause are victims of female fatigue that has a biological basis." No wonder the Latins have siestas.

Keeping in good shape is also a great way to forestall the beginning of what the medical books quaintly call the degenerative diseases, i.e. heart trouble, nerve disorders, arthritis; neoplasms, malignant or otherwise. The low cholesterol diet is only sensible from the forties on, so start fighting the fat and the flab. Vitamin B complex, as well as vitamins A and C, are high on the list of body builders, too.

Outdoor exercise becomes even more important than usual. If you are non-athletic, like me, start walking or gardening or take up yoga, but do something! We can't afford to let all those vigorous types steal a march on us. I lean more towards dancing class and exercises myself, or a good game of pool. Unfortunately, very few of my friends have pool tables and I'm still shy about invading the local pool halls. But give me a few more years and I won't be. That, I find, is the loveliest reward for reaching my forties: a gentle sloughing off of inhibitions.

To return to our symptoms (if and when they appear) some of us get irritable, tired, anxious, have trouble breathing or are plagued with hot flashes. Since I've always been prone to bouts of the first three, I found I was already prepared to do battle in that direction. I keep busy with projects and find that it works wonders. Before I stepped up my writing schedules I used to spend an afternoon a week in a local child care center working with migrant workers' children. We volunteers would feed and change the babies, play with or read to the older ones, change occasional dripping pants and for the children who were interested, I would hold an informal art class. I strongly recommend it for anyone who digs kids, but if coping with children en masse makes you nervous, forget it; you'd only be asking for the butterfly net.

At home I adore redecorating rooms, fixing furniture, sculpting, painting—pictures or rocks—(objects d'art, not for lining the driveway), building a terrace, having a slight bash at gardening—quite against the grain for me—cleaning the cellar—much more fun. I love writing articles for a local newspaper and taking

French lessons once a week. But my favorite pastime of all is entertaining. There is nothing like giving a party to cheer one up. As I am a rather disorganized person, I do things by fits and starts, as the spirit moves me.

Each person can find her own list of projects. I envy my friends who do needlepoint and crewel work. One's loving labors can always be on display to be admired as is not the case with a neat cellar. And my tacky non-blooming garden is the despair of my green- thumbed pals, but we have all (being women and eminently sensible) learned to live with our own shortcomings by now. We'd jolly well better learn in hurry if we haven't, because if we should develop hot flashes, dyspnea (difficulty breathing) or an atrophied vagina and itching (God forbid!), we will have to learn to live with them, too. {As mentioned, this is no longer true.} Fortunately, not for long, because that is when doctors can start using the heavy artillery — hormones. Estrogen, progesterone, and sometimes the male hormone testosterone may be used according to your doctor's judgment. Of these three complaints, luckily the easiest to remedy is the dried-up vagina. A cream or estrogen suppository does the job and your husband's tender affection can once again be appreciated. Once your doctor has assessed your needs in the way of hormone therapy half your battle is won. The other half consists of taking your pills and keeping in touch with him so he can regulate any changes that might pop up. In cases of extreme exhaustion sometimes supplementary thyroid is recommended.

Your gynecologist will become your best friend and favorite magician at this point, so pick a good one.

Easier said than done, but try. Researcher in the field of human reproduction Dr. Maxwell Roland feels that there are three main types of gynecologists — the conservative, the moderate and the liberal. The conservative will not administer sex hormones under any circumstances, believing menopause to be a natural process that one must endure, as did our grandmothers. For those without any annoying difficulties a conservative GYN man could be a happy choice. My sensible older sister who gets the morning meno-grumps, as I do, refuses to take any medication, even aspirin (aspirin is reserved for colds and headaches.) She says serenely, "Good Heavens, I don't need any pills, I just get rid of my hostilities by snapping at the family. It doesn't hurt them and it helps me a lot. They're getting used to it now." Definitely a conservative geared for a conservative doctor. {Gynecologists are now becoming very conservative, as mentioned previously.}

The moderate gynecologist, Dr. Roland continues, is willing to give sex hormones only for definite estrogen deficiency symptoms such as hot flashes and vaginal atrophy and sometimes for osteoporosis (brittle bones.) He generally believes in short-term therapy.

The liberal doctors in this field believe that almost all women can benefit from hormonal-replacement therapy until the day they die. An ounce of prevention is their by-word. So if you know exactly what you want in the way of a doctor you can eliminate a few choices to begin with. {Their philosophies are now changing, or should be.}

Three years ago I was in the hands of a moderate and was very happy until he decided I needed a hysterectomy (the removal of the uterus.) Not will-

30

ing to go under the knife without a second opinion to confirm the first, I consulted another gynecologist. He said the operation was completely unnecessary. There were no tumors, and I was very healthy. He happened to be a conservative, but he was also right, as confirmed by my present doctor who is a liberal. I mention my own case to point out that finding someone with whom you feel comfortable and secure is terribly important. If you prefer a woman gynecologist, for heaven's sake don't torture yourself by going to a male doctor—unless you are a masochist. In that case, go and be happy and God Bless.

I'm dwelling on the physical aspects of the menopause in this chapter so we can all understand the changes our bodies are going through. The mental aspects will come later.

Even if we never get one "hot flash" it is a good idea to know what causes them. They are the end product of the hormone reduction as the follicles stop producing the ovum that triggers the pituitary gland, etc. , etc., as noted in the last chapter. Once everything is off balance and slowing down, sometimes erratic spurts of one of the hormones enter the bloodstream (screwing up the whole system if you'll pardon the expression.) The most startled and shocked by this misbehavior are the blood vessels, which immediately dilate, causing a rush of extra blood to the skin. This causes a rosy glow and a great desire for lots of fresh, cool air. If "hot flashes" caused one to yearn for strawberries out of season or magnums of champagne or a sniff of pot, it would be rather inconvenient, not to say expensive. But since fresh air is still free, we are really very lucky and should enjoy it.

In other words, the average female has little to worry about: physically. The conservative doctors are right when they say that menopause is a normal bodily transition from one life phase to another. Most menopausal women never have any difficulty. For those who do, common sense and the right doctor will alleviate practically all their problems.

Sometimes tumors will form in the uterus, necessitating a hysterectomy. Make sure the operation is needed. A recent survey showed that 28 percent of the hysterectomies performed in Los Angeles were "probably not justified." Hemorrhaging is always a sign that all is not right in one's interior. Run, don't walk to your nearest doctor, after you've mopped up, of course. Women should only trail clouds of glory.

No man yet born will ever understand the possible trauma of a hysterectomy for a woman. On the other hand, women have always known of man's fear of castration, the knowledge of which some women use with devastating effect, like Mrs. Portnoy.

But men, even doctors, will say "what's so special about a hysterectomy? It's just another operation, like an appendectomy." It's all very well for them to say that to us, but if it were a case of whacking off one of their testicles (an orchiectomy) we would hear howls of anguish even after we reassured them that they would lose neither their sex appeal nor their sex life. I could have said "Whose ox is gored now?" but that would have been a bum steer.

A hysterectomy in one's twenties, if one wants to bear children, is very unfortunate, to say the least. But the same operation in one's forties is not a tragedy. Two of my friends who had hysterectomies in their early forties wished they had had it done years before. Both mentally and physically they felt one hundred per cent better. They had always suffered violently from menstrual difficulties which got worse as they grew older. They had also completed their families, one with four children and the other with five. Both are now relaxing and enjoying their husbands' attentions with great enthusiasm. Their energy is boundless and they remain feminine to their fingertips. In their case, the operation was definitely desired, at the same time it solved various problems. They take their supplementary hormones very happily.

Where the operation is not wanted, it becomes a question of cooperating with the inevitable. When one considers that the poor old uterus is doomed in a few years to non-functioning existence, it only makes sense to have it removed if it begins to be a threat to one's health. Men are not all wrong when they superficially liken a hysterectomy to an appendectomy — any sick organ should be taken out if at all possible. What they don't understand is that we all, to some extent, suffer from what Betty Friedan called The Feminine Mystique, a myth-fantasy which tells us we are nothing but walking wombs, among other things. This self-image becomes a stumbling block and should be exorcised at all costs.

Another of my friends who was compelled to have an unwanted hysterectomy zipped around afterwards having lots of affairs to cheer herself up. It perked her up no end, but it sure raised hell with the neighborhood. I wouldn't recommend such a drastic course of action for everyone. Take a trip, get a job, study Swahili or at least have a quiet affair in a strange town, unless, of course, you have masses of understanding friends.

Actually my frisky friend was just doing what comes naturally to an Indian tribe out West. There the social mores are exactly the opposite of ours. The women of the tribe look forward eagerly to the menopause because then their happy duty is to initiate the young bucks into the various rites of love-making. Who wants an inhibited vestal virgin when he can have an experienced pro for free? I can hear the patter of little feet heading west right now.

CHAPTER FIVE

Psychological problems are a good deal harder to cope with than physical ones because it is strictly a do-it-yourself program. I am speaking of the average normal female not the woman who needs special psychiatric assistance. The ones who feel they need help should get it as soon as possible to nip their dilemma in the bud before it grows beyond them.

But it behooves the fairly well adjusted woman (we are all a little crackers in some direction) to understand what her mind is up to during menopause as well as her body. Our modern medicine men have chosen for dark reasons best known to themselves,

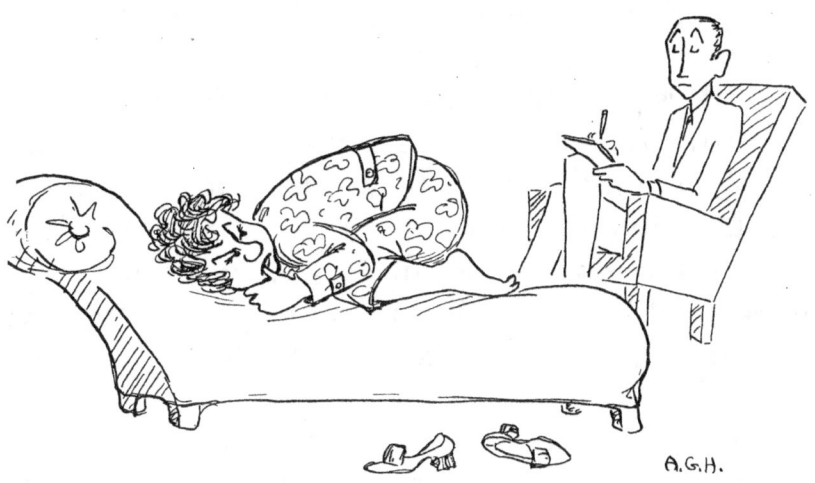

A.G.H.

to call menopause the grand climacteric, opposing it to the menstrual climacteric by which they mean puberty. In point of fact, puberty and menopause are opposite sides of the same coin and display many of the same symptoms, but why that should be so grand defeats me.

A handy fact to know is that there are two parts to menopause. They are the pre-climacteric and the climacteric, and they echo pre-puberty and puberty. The biologic process sends out signals way in advance (literally years) heralding the organic changes to come and these are picked up by our inner spy system. Long before a gynecologist can discover any hormonal imbalance women can start feeling lousy for no apparent reason. Low blood pressure causing abnormal fatigue, and listlessness. General irritability and sleeplessness leading to more of the same. All this sprinkled lavishly with showers of tears. And yet the body is pronounced A-OK on the medical charts. This can really drive you up the wall, as it did me, because then you suspect it must be your mind that is bending, which, of course, it is.

Doctors probably think it is kinder not to let women know they are in for a rather longer siege than expected. Either that, or they don't put two and two together. In any event, once the body receives these signals it doesn't just sit still, it does something about it. Some of the protective measures it takes are to be encouraged and others to be controlled, as best we can.

The body's pre-climacteric struggle puts all the power of ego to work to achieve a better adjustment to reality. Old values tend to take a back seat while a desire to experience something new and exciting takes over. Well channelled, this can be a great boon. The phrase 'The Roaring Forties' isn't just a geographic expression. Our energy returns whether we like it or not and like a boiling tea kettle our excess steam can make wheels go round instead of flipping our lid.

36

Apparently we females are generally divided into three basic types: the motherly, the erotic and the masculine, each of us being mostly one with varying degrees of the other two types thrown in. Our inner attitudes are more or less ruled by which slot we fall into. As the little war drums start beating inside we become more aware of our own persona as an entity and experience a desire to preserve our femininity. This is due to displaced psychic energy, especially if we are at the stage where our children are becoming independent. The emotional void they leave has to be filled in some fashion.

In general, the motherly type of woman has an easy time during menopause if she has been a mother who lets her children go free. The children feeling secure and not strangled by the umbilical cord return to such a woman with their spouses and their own children and resume close family ties that are emotionally rewarding. If she has alienated her offspring a mother can always try a little harder with a late batch or she can put her energies to work outside the home.

It seems that many women in this category have a special talent that they have put aside while rearing their children in fear that it would jeopardize their ability to be a good wife and mother. The smart female either consciously or subconsciously revives this talent in music, art, literature or whatever. Thus the closing of one door only means the opening of another into a new exciting life. That many women do just this automatically shows how powerful our instinct for self-preservation is. The ego, invisible and weightless, works marvels. Sometimes, just before the procreative gates bang shut, the motherly type feels compelled to have more children, sometimes against her conscious will if her psychic power rushes directly to the threatened sector, the womb. This is not helped by the fact that lots of women don't realize that their ovaries can produce hatchable eggs for a whole year after their last period. Something to bear in mind.

With the feminine-erotic woman the ego also cones prancing to the rescue. Freud put it very succinctly when he said, "Love for one's own person is perhaps the secret of beauty." Feminine narcissism seems to be a powerful psychic cosmetic.

Many a beautiful narcissistic woman, whose affairs are beginning to come under the heading of therapy, prepares for menopause long before the first signs again without conscious thought. Filled with a genuine need to be loved and approved of by others, she enters a field of public endeavor like politics or philanthropy or she becomes a patroness of the arts, thus assuring her sense of importance in the world around her. The ego is just as happy with approval of her good works as it was of her beauty, which in point of fact doesn't seem to leave her. Her happy memories of a full, rich past sustain her. The feminine-erotic woman continues her swinging existence unabated.

In some cases the woman who has the easiest menopause is the masculine woman. She has never felt that her personality has depended on her womb-toting state, so the loss of same doesn't threaten her inner stability. Her inclination to compete with males usually leads her to a career of some sort, and if she is happy and successful in her profession she is too busy to pay any attention to either her physical or mental changes. She sails through with a tail wind. Psychiatrists call this intellectual sublimation and to some extent we will all develop good healthy sublimations.

A symptom to be prepared for is a renewed (if we have lost it) interest in sex. This is due both to our psychological feeling of diminishing power and our hormonal activity. Something like this sneaking up on one out of the clear blue sky can be scary but if we are forewarned at least we'll know which way to jump. A jump in the hay can be worth two in the bush, and a lot more comfortable. But for a reserved, strait-laced soul I would suggest taking up golf: having affairs can be very traumatic if you are not geared for them.

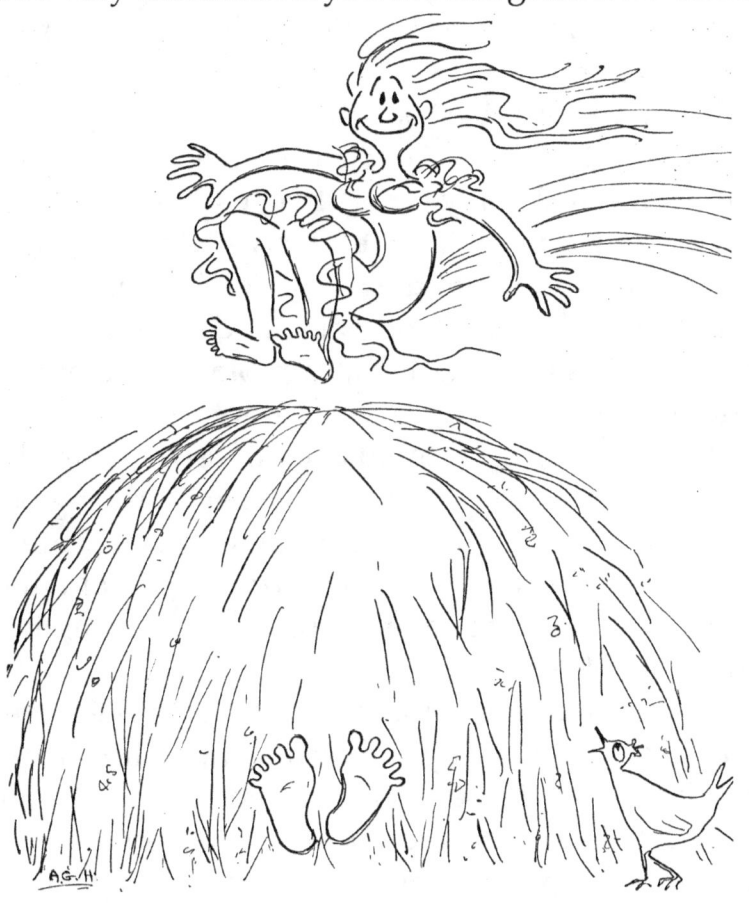

It is the inner struggle against these new sensations that sometimes produce odd behavior patterns. Now is the time to stop calling certain kettles black for what we consider eccentric in others today we may find ourselves doing tomorrow.

Gradually the pre-climacteric changes into the climacteric with all the endocrine imbalances mentioned before: the lessening menstrual periods, etc. As the pressures mount, "some women flee from reality into fantasies, and others from fantasies into reality," according to Helen-Deutsch in The Psychology of Women. This can lead one into the rarified atmosphere of a mystic or ascetic kind. These aren't bad choices either.

What we have to be on guard against are depressed moods and stabs of inferiority feelings. Knowing these are chemically caused helps a little, but not much. Sometimes I think it is just as effective to throw oneself head first into the Slough of Despond when it appears, wallow in it and enjoy one's misery. Tiptoeing around the edges usually prolongs the eventual sinking in the quicksand. Everyone will find her own method of coping, without doubt, for we women are, if nothing else, very ingenious. If we chart our gloomy lows on a calendar we will find they are fairly predictable and many doctors feel that trying to avoid undue stress when we are least prepared to cope with it is only sensible.

Don't have your house guests, a barbecue or a P.T.A. meeting, and a cub scout hike all scheduled for the same weekend. Do spend the afternoon in bed curled up with the novel you haven't had time to read, or slip off to the movies and indulge in popcorn and candies, or go on a shopping bender just for yourself—you can always return the bad mistakes the next day. A helpful thing to remember is that invariably these moods of depression are followed by ones of elation. Pendulum-like, the deeper the despair the higher the elation.

Another important point for our peace of mind is to be reassured about our complete physical health, not just our gynecological well-being. A thorough physical checkup will allay subconscious fears about our heart, lungs, liver and lights. Nagging worries can start a whole chain reaction of psychosomatic symptoms such as headaches, backaches or bellyaches. These we can do without.

If our fundamental need for love, companionship, peer approval and security is thwarted, our emotions are aroused, mobilizing energy for action. The amount of energy created depends on the provocation and can range from minor annoyance to intense anger. In most instances the mobilized energy is expended by direct or indirect action which resolves the problem. It is only when the individual fails to release this excess energy that it becomes a threat to health. Another way to wind up with those famous "psychosomatic symptoms difficult to enquire."

But whatever our type, lessons are to be learned from all three. The motherly female has the gift of establishing warm, personal relationships. This ability may not be inborn in everybody but it can be learned to some extent. A loving circle of family and friends is one of the most rewarding spheres to inhabit. In time of emotional upheaval the strength and solidarity of such a group can be a soothing balm.

From the professional beauty we learn that caring enough about our personal appearance seems to work its own therapy in some mysterious way. Those who really want to stay young will. The adage "God helps those who help themselves" applies here in both the physical and psychological sense. The desire to battle age helps the inner chemistry while it also leads one to take good care of one's body, to exercise, eat properly and not overindulge in the savory goodies of life like alcohol and tobacco. I was going to add sex, but none of the books I've read have put it on the no-no list. In fact, Dr. David Reuben in his Everything You Always Wanted to Know About Sex implies that vigorous sexual activity forestalls heart attacks, hardening of the arteries and arthritis. Certainly an interesting theory to try to prove, if you are so inclined.

The example of the successful professional woman is especially significant. As Helene Deutsch puts it, "Almost every woman in the climacteric goes through a shorter or longer phase of depression. While the active women deny the biologic state of affairs, the depressive ones overemphasize it." Since we are talking about troubles that start in our head, what better way to short-circuit our apprehensions than to never let them start.

A large percentage of these anxieties stem from our basic fear of growing older. Everyone gets hoist by her own petard sooner or later. The first wrinkles and puckers of our thirties warn us that there is such a thing as age; something no one believes, concerning themselves in their twenties. What we are engaged in is simply the same old war against aging. We have become the front line troops in a battle which turns out to be not a battle or even a skirmish, but just a delaying action while we negotiate with our old enemy: time. Grab your weapons, fire at will, keep firing and don't fall back. We have nothing to lose but our gray hair.

CHAPTER SIX

Now that we know what is going on inside our bodies and minds during menopause and basically what to do about it (Well, we do, don't we?) let's look at how some of our fellow females have coped using the same equipment; equipment doled out to all of us by our Creator with glorious impartiality. The easiest people to spot, of course, are the ones who make the news. Articles with photographs tell and show us every day that growing older can also mean growing more attractive.

I remember going to the theatre about ten years ago with my husband. We were sitting in a box and to amuse ourselves were picking out the two most beautiful women we could see. My turn was first and I chose a young, fresh-faced, straight-haired blond with even New England features. My husband was less than impressed. "She looks dull as hell to me!" He grabbed the opera glasses, swept the orchestra and pointed like a bird dog to a dark haired girl seated in a middle row. "Now that's what I call a real beauty! She looks just like Loretta Young used to when I saw her in Hollywood back in '33."

I had to admit he was right. The stunning brunette made my choice seem insipid, with or without the glasses. After the entr'acte my husband, who is a born prowler, came back from the lobby wearing an extremely pleased expression. "I told you I could pick them. That *is* Loretta Young and she looks even better close up." Today Miss Young is in her early sixties and I know jolly well that my husband would still point like a bird dog.

People have their own self-image that they live up to; an inner myth that sustains them. (A myth being a vehicle of communication between the conscious and the unconscious.) Performers have the added ability to change their self-images at will; that is what they have been trained for. One minute, earth-mother, the next seductress, innocent ingénue or eccentric aunt. This talent for adjustment is formidable to say the least as it rests on a strong ego allowing them to move

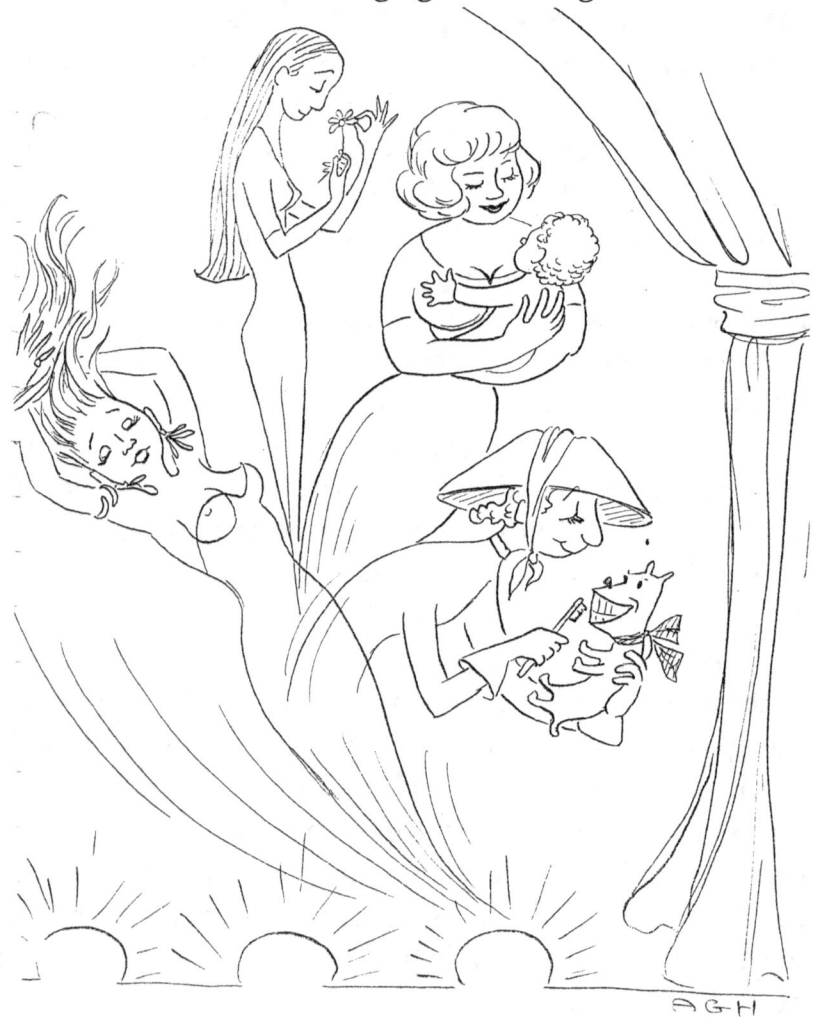

in any direction with complete security. They do with their personalities what a dancer does with her or his body; the extremities always moving out from a perfectly balanced inner core or corps, if you will. That is why I feel actresses can age so charmingly. They are continually growing, learning and greeting new experiences with enthusiasm. Performers like Angela Lansbury, forty-seven; Lauren Bacall, forty-eight and Alexis Smith, forty-nine, returned to New York to give smash performances in musicals; something new for all of them. Their freshly trained aching muscles were worth it, as Broadway turned somersaults. Fifty years and older like Peggy Lee, Lena Home, Ingrid Bergman, Pearl Bailey, Lucille Ball and sixty-year oldsters like Katherine Hepburn, Joan Crawford, Bette Davis, Arlene Francis and Marlene Dietrich are still packing whatever theatres are lucky enough to get them. {In this century this list would include such dynamic women as Meryl Streep, Susan Sarandon, Helen Mirren and Dame Judy Dench. {(Dame Edna, as brilliant as she is, doesn't qualify.)}

Just as good generals do, all these women operate from positions of power and I refer to inner power which might even be called a state of grace, if one wants to get metaphysical.

But is it just women trained professionally to lock horns with life who can stir up the dust on the middle plateau? Hardly. Take for instance a fat (214 lb.) talkative Queens, NY housewife who could have kept eating busily through her forties, wishing vainly that she were thinner and life were more exciting. She didn't. Instead Mrs. Jean Neiditch put her gift of gab together with her desire to lose weight and started

Weight Watchers, now a multi-million dollar international organization with franchises in England, Australia, West Germany and Israel. At forty-eight Mrs. Neiditch weighs in at 142 pounds, is worth almost six million and is very attractive indeed. A real nifty job of image changing while living off the fat of the land.

An Urbana, Illinois housewife named Natalie Alpert became a landscape architect in her forties, graduating from the University of Illinois the same year that her youngest daughter graduated from Stanford. She started from scratch to earn her B.A., first one course, then school half time, then full time, as she came down the home stretch. Her family was behind her every inch of the way, her daughters teaching her math and her husband kindly ignoring her somewhat sketchy housekeeping while cheering her on.

In Atlanta, Georgia, housewife Marylin Davis parleyed her legal secretarial expertise and volunteer political activities into a job as administrative assistant to a stockbroker. After intensive study she passed the New York Stock Exchange examination for a license and is now a full-fledged stock broker practicing in a very tough field for females to crack. Her husband finds her more interesting than ever. The husband of New Jersey-ite Leonore Berck finds his wife a more exciting companion too, for she has used her knowledge of music and running music and arts groups for charity to land a job as cultural arts director of the Bergen County Y.M. and Y.W.H.A. One would almost think that all these women had hired Alan Lakein's time management consultant firm as does I.B.M. and The Bank of America. But I'm sure all of them have done intuitively what Mr. Lakein charges $50 an hour to teach to harassed businessmen.

First they have defined their lifetime goals, then they have defined their five-year goals, and through careful planning and concentrated effort have given their lives a full, rounded form, working as a sculptor does, minute by minute, day by day, until at last the whole figure is complete. Lakein feels that a five- year plan gives a sense of motion and potential. As my sister said when she started studying for her PhD at age forty-four, "I might just as well be forty-nine with a doctorate as without one."

Instead she fell madly in love with a middle-aged fellow student for the first time in her life, got married, and promptly got pregnant. A spinster school teacher who didn't know she was the motherly type

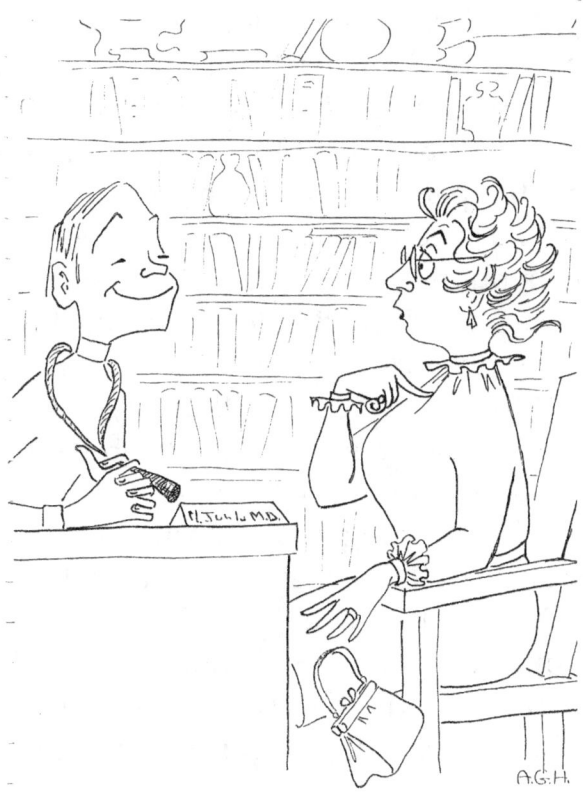

but who very happily changed not only her five year plan but her life plan to include a beautiful blue-eyed daughter. Mr. Lakein might tear his hair out over that case, but my sister certainly doesn't lack any sense of motion or potential as anyone with a seven year old around the house knows.

A case that would have Mr. Lakein purring like a cream-fed kitten would be a friend of mine whose life has fallen into very happy patterns, not exactly by accident. She once said to me, "I've been so lucky all my life, every ten years I've had something new and exciting happen. At twenty I was singing with Paul Whiteman's orchestra. I was good too. At thirty I had written some very successful children's books and had a great career as an editor going. At forty I remarried and my husband and I started our own publishing company. At fifty I discovered that I could sculpt and I love it. I'm good at that, too. I can't wait to find out what happens when I reach sixty. I know it will be great." It has been, too, because she and her husband sold their publishing house for a nice profit, moved to London and are having loads of fun starting a new publishing business from scratch.

I don't for a minute think that any of this just happened: that life presented my friend with a super Christmas present every ten years. There was lots of hard work, planning and determination behind all the "good luck." She may have had what social scientist, Dr. Orville Brim, Jr. calls a "middle years... continuing discontent with one's self, a day-to-day self-appraisal and a continuing search for self-esteem," but if she did, the feeling was used as a goad not a crutch.

50

My super-charged friend didn't need Mr. Lakein to tell her how to handle her time. In fact none of us need pay $50 an hour to have an expert tell us that we all have "untouched pockets of creativity" or that "without imagination there can be no alternatives and no motivation." We have known this from the day we were born and if it slips our minds sometimes it is only because we've been too busy keeping house or keeping jobs or raising children to concentrate on our inner selves. But, now like Luis Borges, we can say

...I reach my center,
my algebra and my key,
my mirror.
Soon I shall know who I am.

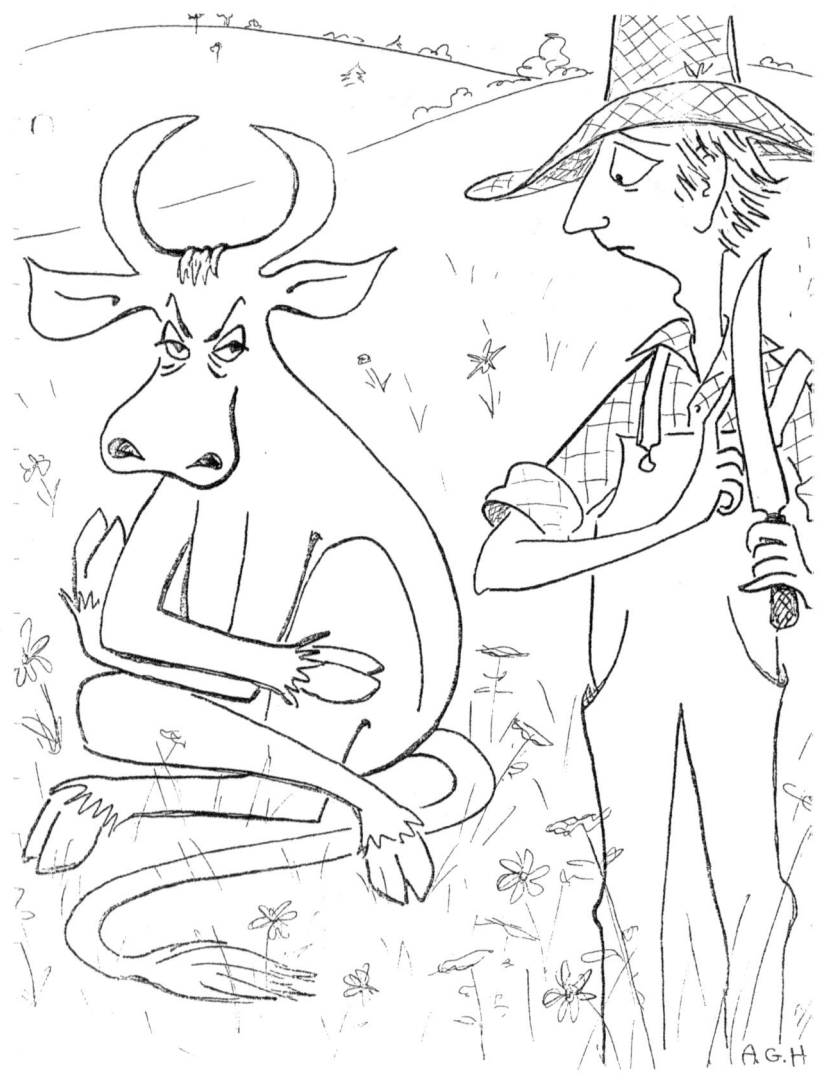

CHAPTER SEVEN

Let's tackle a very elusive subject indeed — male menopause. It is apt to cause women as much trouble as men, and yet medical books barely mention it. Could male chauvinism be rearing its beaming countenance? No matter; like the pyramids, it is there.

Testosterone is to men what estrogen is to women: the main sex hormone. It governs their primary and secondary sexual characteristics — primary being their desire for, and amount of, sexual activity and secondary being the physical manifestations of maleness; beard, heavy muscles, long bones, aggressive behavior, all of which the Greeks wrap up in a lovely word, machismo.

Once scientists had determined that testosterone was the key to male's sexuality they couldn't wait to get their hands on some to experiment with. No simple task. Poor old Ernst Laqueur had to process nearly a ton of bulls' testicles to render less than one-hundredth of an ounce of pure testosterone crystals. No matter how you slice it, that's a lot of bull.

It is the imperceptible lessening of the amount of testosterone in the bloodstream that causes male menopause. This starts at age 50 or 55 and goes on for years and years. They, of course, don't notice it as there are no lessening periods to watch for or hot flashes to endure, except in very rare cases.

The endocrine system of the male is very similar to that of the female. The pituitary gland is the big cheese who gives the orders, but in the male's case it sends the messages down to the testes instead of the ovaries. The signals are carried by gonadtropic hormones, one of which is called ISCH (Interstitial cell stimulating hormone.) It is similar to the females (LH) and is actually called LH by doctors to simplify things. Another hormone is the masculine form of our old friend FSH. The job of the male's LH is to stimulate the Leydig cells into making testosterone. The male FSH hormone wings in on the seminiferous tubules which are the sperm makers. Thus as Dr. Maxwell Roland says, because the female has only one tissue to produce both her germ cells (eggs) and her female hormones, once her ovaries are shot menopause sets in. On the other hand, since the male has two sets of tissues, (one for his sperm and another for his male hormones) the male has the benefit of sex hormones for twenty years longer than the female.

Men's interior endocrine game is more like a cricket match than a baseball game. Once the hormonal activity starts at puberty it rocks along very evenly for sixty or seventy years. The signals are given in quiet, well modulated tones, sometimes the Sertoli cells informing the pituitary that "a shade too much FSH in that last bowl, old boy" and the pituitary murmuring politely, "Dreadfully sorry; bit too much wrist, I expect." The automatic signal exchange only slows down when the players begin to age and take a little longer at bat. But slow down it does. This gradual diminishing production of testosterone by the Leydig cells plus possible eccentric behavior by the pituitary (and the thyroid and adrenal glands, if they are unlucky) changes both the male body and psyche. The physiological changes are almost imperceptible. It is the psychological changes that create merry hell if they pop up. The fact that most men are blessed with no ill effects whatsoever has given rise to the myth of the non-menopausal male. Thus the poor men who are affected are ill prepared. Like little lost lambs they run around getting into nothing but trouble. Trouble being mostly women and more women, sometimes with a little gambling and booze thrown in to sweeten the pot.

Up until their fifties most men feel young and virile; their careers are humming along and their home life represents security even if it isn't perfect. Then zap — the half-century mark and fifteen years until retirement. Their options seem to be melting away and they wonder if they have really done all the things that they wanted to do with their lives. This can lead to a job identity crisis. I am sure this is what psychoanalyst Erik Erikson had in mind when he said, "In some periods of his history, and in some phases of his life cycle, man needs a new ideological orientation as surely and sorely as he must have air and food." Sane men sublimate their powerful feelings of unrest successfully. Others become neurotic and others take their courage in both hands and strike out in a completely new direction. A man I know who is in his latish forties found out that he really hated banking and wanted to work in the advertising field. Having a gung-ho wife and kids solidly behind him helped him make the decision to change jobs and location in one fell swoop. Another friend left the gray-flannelled ranks of Madison Avenue to strike out on his own as a portrait painter. They are both much happier in their new lives. God forbid I should call these men menopausal. It just happened that their job identity crisis arrived close to the magic age of 50. This can as easily happen to career women as to men, and obviously causes an equal amount of anguish. Unfortunately if these feelings of general discontent hit a husband really hard after the half century mark this is usually the time when the man's poor wife, having finished her siege of menopause, is relaxed and off-guard. She feels her marriage of twenty or thirty years is secure, so the hell with face creams, diets and exercises — let 'er rip. Hair curlers, flannel nightgowns and a razor-sharp tongue can become her weapons of self-destruction.

The male, inarticulate in his longing for his lost youth begins to search for ways to recapture it. If the home front is unattractive, over the fence and into greener fields he goes full tilt.

The husband may take up dieting where his wife left off. Extra games of tennis or golf keep him trim and prove the old muscles still zing. Younger looking clothes may make their appearance, topped off by a hair piece. Woe betide the wife who makes fun of any of these signs. Since we all expect endless amounts of sympathy and understanding during our climacteric we had jolly well better be prepared to offer gobs of said commodities to our suffering spouses. Alfred Kinsey pointed out in his weighty tome that 85% of the total sexual outlet of married males is confined to their wives. Lucky us. But the kicker is that half of all married men sleep with other women during their marriage. (Little grabsies in the pantry don't count.) So what we don't know about has probably already happened.

As in our case, the hormonal imbalance in the bloodstream plus the dreaded aging process lurking

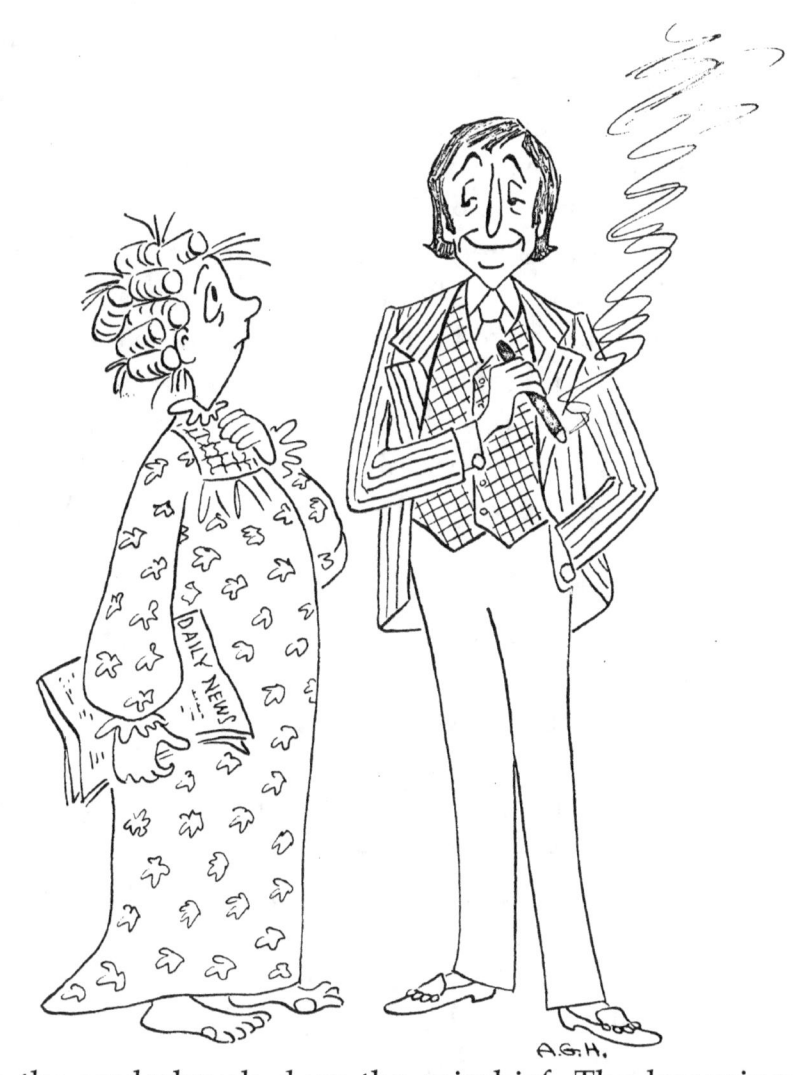

in the underbrush does the mischief. The lessening amount of testosterone in the system slows down the male's sexual activity and if he is the type to panic, he will. A new bed companion or a series of them will temporarily titillate tired glands, a fact that can turn a Casper Milquetoast into a leering prancing billy-goat. Since men are more highly geared erotically than women, get satisfaction quicker, need a greater variety of stimuli and experimentation, they can easily find themselves between a rock and a hard place, as the Southerners would say.

If they have read the Kinsey Report they know the dismal news that at age 55 about 8% of all white males have become impotent. After 55 the number of unfortunates increases rapidly. By 75 more than one-half of all white males have had it sexually. The Negro male fares better; sometimes staying potent until 80, and one lively 88 year old Black on record was still having regular intercourse with his 90-year-old wife. Black is beautiful in more ways than one. {Nowadays Viagra and other medications take care of most of these problems.}

The unfortunate male who does suffer menopausal symptoms can suffer a slew of them, just like us. It's a long list; read it and weep.

1. Extreme nervousness
2. Tension to the extent of tremulousness; otherwise known as the shakes
3. Lack of concentration due to slowed down mental processes
4. Depression
5. A feeling of futility
6. Loss of self confidence
7. Lassitude
8. Vague pains in various parts of the body
9. Sleeplessness

Any poor bastard who hits the big jackpot develops a classic dose of involutional melancholia or "climacteric psychosis." As if that isn't enough, the misbegotten waifs can get upset tummies and constipation, too, which doesn't seem fair, somehow. Not to mention "formication," a sensation of insects crawling over the skin. Watch how you pronounce that one. As a matter of fact, we women can get formication, too, though I hate to mention it.

One thing the menopausal male has going for him is a vast amount of literature written solely with his problem in mind. For those tired glands there are the girlie magazines including and especially Playboy. {The computer has provided access to pornography, also.} On a different plane we have a plethora of novels about restless middle-aged men with job and/or marriage crises. To quote one New York Times book review of April, 1972, about The Landlocked Man, "Mr. Coppel's novel is the sequel to all those books in which the hero kicks over his job at the ad agency to go up to Vermont and write.... But Robert Martin, 50-year-old ex-creative director of F. A. Green Associates, cannot write finis to the rat race.... Martin has adopted something akin to the Protestant work ethic toward Christy Petersen, the 23-year-old admirer who shares his cabin." In the same issue we see a two-column ad for an autobiography called A Letter to my Wife, by John B. Koffend. It reads in part, "John Koffend entered middle age with a lot going for him. A good job as an editor at Time Magazine, a fine family and a love affair so satisfying that he had planned to divorce his wife of nineteen years to marry the woman he truly loved." This vicarious living through other people's problems in print is to the male what a juicy soap opera is to a female, so why knock it.

What do you do if your best beloved seems to be getting a bit restive? The psychiatrists have discovered that the strongest factor in any marriage is a determination that it shall endure. The individual makes her or himself put up with a lot of jazz that would otherwise cause a smash up. The Catholic Church has known this for centuries. So the first thing you do is make your mind up firmly that you will hang on by your teeth no matter what.

Concerning extra-marital affairs, Anna Kleegman says in The Mature Woman: Her Richest Years, "The wise wife will ignore her mate's occasional lapses during this period, knowing, if she faces the situation realistically, that they do not mean anything unless she allows them to mean something...the clever woman will not permit wounded pride or vanity to destroy her entire lifework."

The second thing to do is to take a long, hard look at yourself and see if you like what you see. Are you really as attractive as you could be, or as thoughtful or as much fun? No man in his right mind will stray far from a charming, loving mate. At least not for long. And one of the most loving things you could do is convince the man in your life that he should see a urologist and get some shots of testosterone. Good dollops of this male hormone will do for him what estrogen does for us. Dr. Robert Greenblatt has used hormone therapy for his male patients for years and says of them, "most have reported a return of vigor and vitality; they are convinced that they feel better, work more effectively, and get more enjoyment out of life."

You might also invest in a few marriage manuals to find some exotic ideas about how to surprise your husband in bed. You will know much better than I just how much surprise he can take: Man is really a tender creature who should be cosseted. Spoil him rotten and you have him for life. Keep calling him a son-of-a-bitch and he's going to be somebody else's son-of-a-bitch in no time flat. If you are the kind that goes all out then be like George Simenon's wife who allows her husband complete sexual freedom and can serenely pack their suitcases in a hotel suite while Simenon gets four successive chicks in the sack next door.

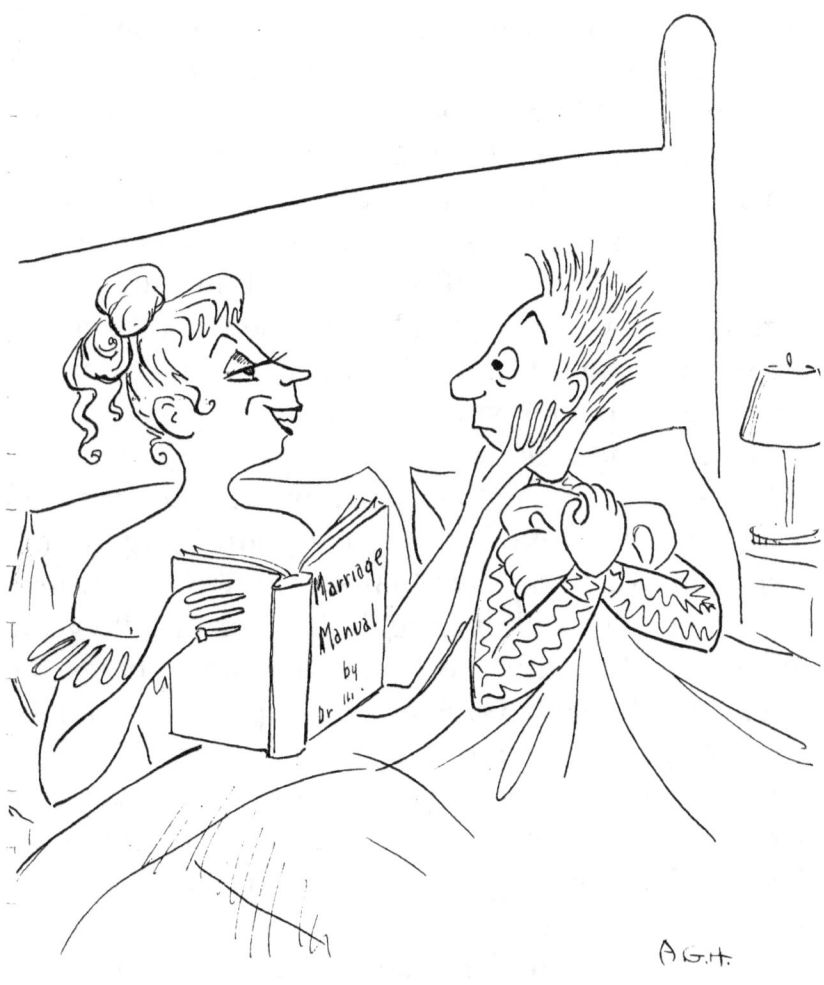

A.G.H.

Dr. Ruben expounds a lovely theory in his new book Any Woman Can. It concerns how to catch a man, but could just as easily apply to how to keep a man. Man's four basic needs are food, sex, love and individual identity. For the infant at his mother's breast all these needs are satisfied. Milk, even from a bottle assumes an almost magical power over the male that lasts all his life. So unless it is off his diet, ply your other half (I very carefully didn't say better half in mute salute to the Woman Libbers) with lots of milk in any form; ice cream, milk shakes, hot chocolate, homemade bread, cookies or candy, etc. And if you can possibly manage to feed him a few bites by hand that will really lasso his wandering psyche.

You have another thing going for you with food and that is its aphrodisiac qualities. The German nutritionist Dr. Hans Balzli swears that all humankind is more susceptible to the blandishments of the opposite sex after a perfect meal than at any other time. In short, you can cook yourself into ecstasy — or stir the pot and hit the sack.

It is a very healthy theory in any event so what can you lose? Even if you gain a few pounds, a psychiatrist friend of mine says that some men fall in love with their wives all over again in their middle years and especially with the things a woman hates the most about herself; wrinkles, excess poundage, all the signs of age she tried to conceal.

Don't ask me the explanation for that one. Since it is a man-made theory I'm not even sure I quite believe it. Those ivory tower boys come up with some weirdies now and again.

Dr. Reuben, on the other hand, can usually be

trusted with good horse sense. One of the most sensible things he recommends is that any woman should provide her man with "an inexhaustible supply of reassurance and consolation." If you can convince him that he is the most uniquely perfect person who has ever graced your presence, the battle is won. Obviously No one else in the whole wide world will ever tell him that.

I trust that if you follow all this advice very carefully you'll never have any trouble with your husband (or lover) whatsoever. On the other hand, he may run off howling into the wilderness. Those are the chances you take, but since any cat, be it tabby or tom, prefers a warm place where it gets three squares a day and can curl up and get its belly rubbed, I think your chances are good.

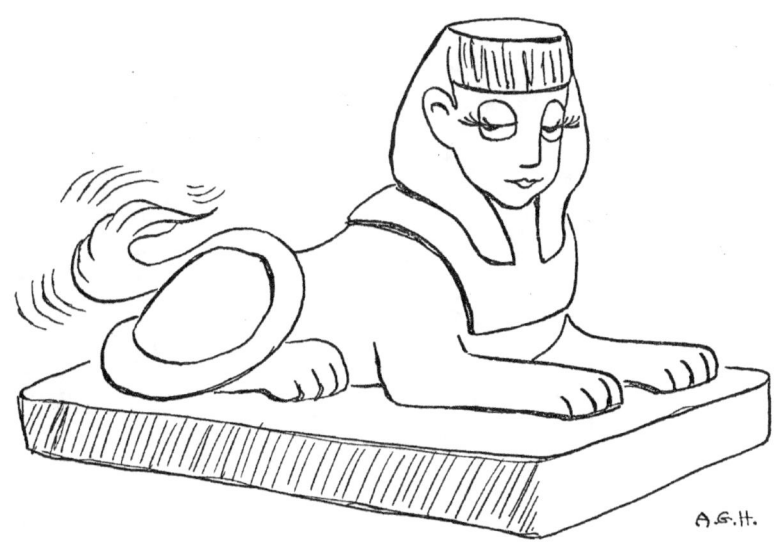

CHAPTER EIGHT

And now dear hearts and constant readers, I bear glorious news. Each and every one of us is indeed "The Eternal Woman." I have this from no less an authority than Buckminster Fuller—noted scientist, philosopher, mathematician, inventor, poet and writer, whose giant geodesic dome housed the U.S. exhibition at Canada's Expo '70. His revolutionary plans for feeding and housing the earth's population have fascinated Russians, the Japanese, the Canadians, the Indians—in fact the whole world. He is kept on the hop conferring with worried heads of state everywhere.

Bucky Fuller's thought patterns are unique and very complex, but since he is a devoted admirer of womankind, they are well worth delving into, so pull up your panty-hose and concentrate.

His theory starts out simply enough with tension and compression. They coexist in all things and always abide by their inbuilt laws. Kids might say "pull" and "squeeze". If you pull a knotted rope taut the knot will become "squeezed" or compressed tighter and its girth will contract. (If you are curious it compresses in a plane at 90 degrees to its tensed axis, so there.)

If you consider an object controlled by compression you will find that short, fat columns or pillars are stronger than long, thin ones. If you've ever wondered why it is because "the structural capabilities of columns loaded in compression reach an early limit of what is known as their slenderness ratio, i.e. the relationship between the column's girth diameter and its length." (Mr. Fuller added, when he read the chapter for accuracy, "If your reader thinks that it doesn't

65

apply to everyday life, tell them that man has developed his sensitivities so highly that he can judge the slenderness ratio of any woman's legs within a 64th of an inch from 100 yards away.")

On the other hand the opposite is true of a cable, an object controlled by tension. It has "no fundamental slenderness limit of ratio of length in respect to girth diameter ... due to its having a no limit tensional-slenderness ratio. This trend approaches very great length with zero girth diameter." It may seem odd to think of an invisible cable (zero girth diameter) having great strength until we realize "that the moon and earth are tensionally cohered by gravity." This is true of all of the celestial bodies in the universe.

(Again I was fixed by what must be the largest, most perceptive eyes in the world.) "You should indicate here the fantastic strength of this invisible cable. The pull of the moon on the earth, 3/4 of which is covered by water, is equal to" — here he pulled out an old envelope and started figuring. Minutes later he finished. "The moon lifts approximately one quintillion tons of water approximately five feet daily. This energy used every day makes the combined atomic stockpile of both Russia and the United States look like one frail snow crystal in the Himalaya Mountains." He added, "A propros of your book, the moon-pull also gives women their menstrual tensional coherence to the moon."

To return to our stubby column, if we shorten and fatten it enough it will become a sphere and the sphere is "nature's optimum limit in structural opposition to compressive forces ... ergo, the stars and the planets and atoms are all spherical islands of compression."

66

Here is where we females begin to tiptoe into the picture although you may not suspect it—but—"nature employs discontinuous compressions and continuous tension. For this reason, compressions are plural and tension is singular."

We women are tensional and continuous; i.e. Eternal because "each new female as well as male life comes from the womb of the woman. We have, then, the new female life as a series of expanding waves, the new ever emerging from within the older wave. Women are thus continuous, like the single-cell creature, Hydra, the newer part breaking off from the older with its early life overlapping its mother's later life—ergo, never dying. Males are discontinuous. The new life is non-continuous to the previous male life. Men are, then, islanded individual discontinuities.

(Mr. Fuller added, "Man was in woman, but woman was not in man—man continues to return into woman to keep universe going.")

At any rate, the next time you get mad at your husband or whomever, instead of the usual Anglo-Saxon expletive, call him an "islanded individual discontinuity" and see what happens. Probably a lot of continual tension, but it's worth a try.

So there we females are, tense and eternal, which makes us little powerhouses of hidden energy. We never use most of it but the small part we do makes us potent indeed. It is our tensional quality that makes us attractive, in its literal sense, to males. Mr. Fuller's theory is that we employ tension "as does a trout angler, on a long invisibly thin flexible line whose slackening allows the male to play himself out darting hither and yon, while being gradually reeled in where

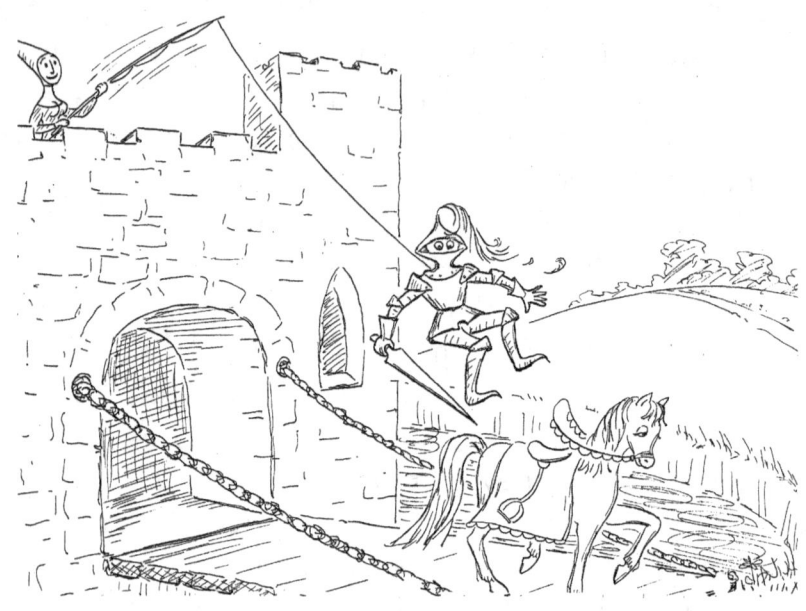

he finally flops into the boat and into bed."

As if this were not enough ego-food for one day, Fuller points out that all through history we women have been the conservers of food and clothing, the organizers of the home crew to perform necessary life-tasks, and the inventors of better ways of food storage and weaving, etc. Man was the hunter who roamed about preying on animals, while we women stayed back at the hearth. When man returned with a new prize, "woman had to decide whether to kill it, skin it or milk it."

We then designed the necessary implements needed, such as baskets, flasks, needles, etc. for these necessities, consolidating all these gains while keeping the home fires burning and rearing our children. We literally invented industry, which was only pried from our grasp when men acquired enough spare time between tribal wars to sit around the hearth, brood, and then start turning woman's industry into trade. Once man busied himself with better production of — and markets for — his goods, woman began to take a back seat. We have been back-seat drivers ever since. Even today, controlling as we do the ownership shares of great industries, we keep our mouths shut, "The Solid Gold Cadillac," notwithstanding.

Another fact that Mr. Fuller points out is that although today the majority of humans alive are pre-menopausal, by the end of the century the center of gravity in the relative age of population will shift from pre-menopausal to post-menopausal. The leveling-off of the birth rate in the industrial countries plus the lengthening life span are the reasons for the transition. At any rate, our generation will be the spearhead of a new lifestyle for the majority of humankind, which gives one pause for thought. All men and women alike have a chance now to be truly creative, a deliciously drunk-making idea. Up until now mankind has stubbornly backed into the future, ass-backwards as it were, with his eyes firmly glued to the past. But we are finally leaving this "womb of permitted ignorance" and not a second too soon. The Women's Liberation Movement has begun to unleash woman power, willy-nilly, whether we like it or not. We'd better use it.

H.L. Mencken spotted this trend back in 1918 when he wrote In Defense of Women. Fulsome and flowery, his prose nevertheless carries much the same message as Bucky Fuller's. A small example. "That it should still be necessary, at this late stage in senility of the human race to argue that women have a fine and fluent intelligence is surely an eloquent proof of the defective observation, incurable prejudice and general imbecility of their lords and masters. No shy man with words was Mr. Mencken.

His theory is that any man worth his salt has a "wide streak of woman in him" because we are more perceptive, less sentimental, difficult to deceive and just as bright. He quotes W. L. George who said, "Human creatures are never entirely male or entirely female: there are no men, there are no women, but only sexual majorities."

Mencken believed that some of the supermen (those with a dash of woman in their makeup) of history were Bonaparte, Goethe, Schopenhauer, Lincoln, and Shakespeare. I don't mind keeping that company at all.

To be fair to our "islanded individual discontinuous" friends, I must admit that the reverse is also true. Psychologists believe that a good dollop of male is often the saving grace of many a female. It is an inner core of stability that saves us from smashing ourselves to smithereens on the rocky vicissitudes of life. If I am beginning to sound Menckenish, it is just because I am still getting used to being a tensionally continuous sexual majority who is breasting her way into the future.

CHAPTER NINE

While we are peering at various perspectives of our-selves — and what subject is more intriguing — it might be amusing to cast a side glance back through history to see what we have been. From the be-ginning women have played every role conceivable up to the hilt: virtuous and wanton goddesses in all religions, despotic rulers, brawny-armed warriors, seductive slave-girls, sacrificing mothers or drudges in the kitchen and field. You name it, we did it. Now a pawn — now a potentate, we have run the gamut like a yo-yo.

If, as is postulated by many psychologists, some of our insecurities stem from penis-envy it must also be true that some of men's problems stem from womb-envy. The vicious circle is then completed by our plac-ing undue importance on our own procreative ability because men do.

Like so many other things, the Greeks had a word for it. The Greek men were convinced that women's unstable mental conditions were due to the wan-dering about of the womb inside the body, so they dreamed up lots of catchy ways of restraining it. Fe-male's flighty mental seizures were dubbed "hys-teria," coming from the word "hystera," meaning womb. So if you become hysterical at the thought of a hysterectomy, it's only fitting and proper.

The Greek myths have been scrutinized by all and sundry searchings for basic race-memory and intui-tive insights into psychology and sociology. What struck me was how many times the womb was by-passed in the mythical creation of a new deity, thus downgrading what men did not possess.

Take Zeus, with his mighty migraine asking the local blacksmith, Hephaestus, to cure his headache with an axe blow. Reluctantly the smith does as bidden and out pops Athene, fully armed for battle. Zeus not only ignores Excedrin, but any fooling around with sexual organs, male or female, in producing Athene.

This tendency is inherited by Athene herself, according to Apollodorus. He writes that later Athene asks Hephaestus to forge some arms for her. The blacksmith, having just been ditched by Aphrodite, develops an instant mad lech for Athene. He springs at her. The goddess, a dedicated virgin, will have none of it and flees, hotly pursued by lame Hephaestus. Determination almost makes up for lack of agility but not quite, for by the time the smith catches Athene he (to quote Apollodorus) "discharged his seed on her leg. The disgusted goddess wiped the seed away with some wool and threw it on the ground."

Believe it or not, out of that mess appeared her son Erichthonius.

The greatest look-ma-no-womb story must be the birth of the smithy's ex-flame, the Goddess Aphrodite. It seems that Gaea (Earth) got tired of Uranus's (Sky's) insatiable sexual demands; the silly girl. Gaea gave their son a huge sharp sickle and with it dastardly instructions. Just as weary Uranus sank down for his nightly fun and, games, out jumped Chronos, who with a lethal swing, castrated his old man. He pitched the offending member over his shoulder into the sea where it floated away creating white sea foam out of which arose the beautiful Aphrodite. How does that grab you?

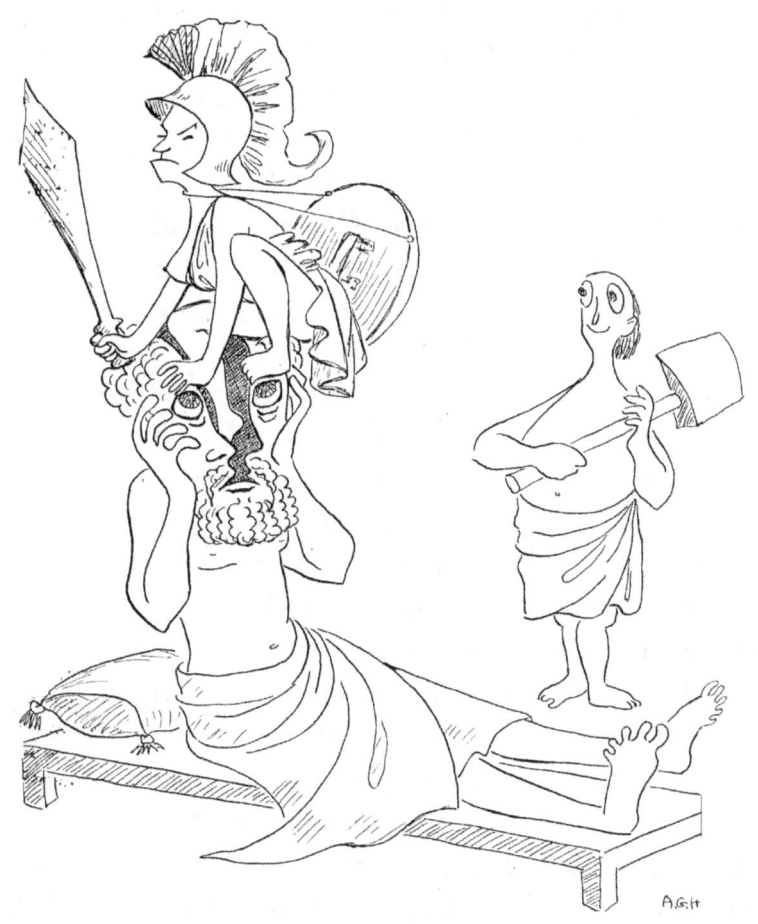

Whatever myth-maker dreamed up that tale must have suffered from both penis and womb-envy, no hermaphrodite, he!

There are many more such bizarre non-births in the myths to attest to the ancient Greeks' jealousy of woman's procreative powers. However they were not only jealous of us but they were scared of us, too.

The Greeks called our periodic bleeding "catharsis" because we were being purged of impurities. Their less learned ancestors would have bluntly said we were discharging evil spirits for we were assumed to have magical faculties during that time. No wonder that we still secretly fear a loss of power after menstruation ceases. All savage peoples have eyed us females with great suspicion once every month; and today civilized peoples do so with only slightly less alarm. Witness Hubert Humphrey's personal physician, Dr. Edgar Berman who made the crack about women being limited in their leadership potential by physiological and psychological factors, especially during the menstrual cycle and menopause. We all bear psychic scars from long centuries of such baleful scrutiny.

At least great affairs of state don't hang on the appearance or non-appearance of our monthly periods as they did for Queen Elizabeth I. It was not the question of her becoming pregnant (The doctors had decided the likelihood of that was nil; virgin queen or no), but the question of making sure her wonky interior continued to function in some way so that she could remain in the marriage market. As long as the general public didn't know the queen was barren the balance of power could be stabilized between her enemies. Foreign suitors like Catherine de Medici's son, the Duke of Anjou (later Henry, III of France), could be kept dangling to keep King Philip, II of Spain nervous. Or if France or Mary Stuart seemed to be threatening, one of Philip, II's Hapsburg cousins could be approached for marriage negotiations. Elizabeth's fair body was dangled now here—now there, for years while England grew strong and her navy supreme.

Shrewd Good Queen Bess was a consummate statesman and politician in every field, even in public relations. Reviewing the troops of Tillway while the dread Spanish Armada ranged off the English coast, Queen Elizabeth said to the people gathered there: "I know I have the body of a weak and feeble woman, but I have the heart and stomach of a king, and of a king of England, too...." With guts like that, who needs a womb?

On the other hand, lack of fecundity ruined Josephine's marriage to Napoleon. Josephine's daughter Hortense wrote in her memoirs about their many trips to Plombiers to take the waters in hopes of curing Josephine's gynecological problems. Hortense was the Empresses' daughter by a previous marriage to the Viscount Beauharnais.

Poor beautiful Josephine: with the onset of menopause, her goose was cooked, and in 1809 when she was 46, Napoleon divorced her to marry Princess Marie-Louise of Austria. History doesn't record whether Josephine cried out at the news of the birth of Marie-Louise's son the way Queen Elizabeth cried out when hearing of the birth of Mary Stuart's son.

However sad her life after the divorce, the ex-Empress kept her charm and beauty intact. Her cosmetic case is still at Malmaison in her dressing room. It is a beautifully inlaid wooden box, the size of a small trunk, jam-packed with jars of creams, unguents, powders, rouges, etc. Judging from a painting done of her in 1813 by Isabey when she was 50, all the creams were worth it, as she looks ravishing.

Women's Lib could take a leaf from Josephine's book now that they have banned the bra. The next step would be to reintroduce the Empire evening gown in sheer see-through cloth, then dampen it the way Josephine and her friends did when they were young. After that, it's every man for himself.

History is filled with women who were prisoners of their uterine canal in one way or another. The brilliant intellectual nymphomaniac, Catherine the Great of Russia, was a happy prisoner indeed, for she had an endless supply of husky young men to feed her greedy appetite.

Sexual freedom has been an off-again, on-again situation for us females down through the ages. The Roman women in 195 B.C. raised hell until they got the *Lex Oppia* changed. This was a law forbidding woman to own more than half an ounce of gold, to use a carriage in Rome — or any provincial town or to wear clothes of many colors.

Cato, after complaining bitterly about women slipping from the authority of their parents, brothers or husbands, goes on to describe in horror their very ac-

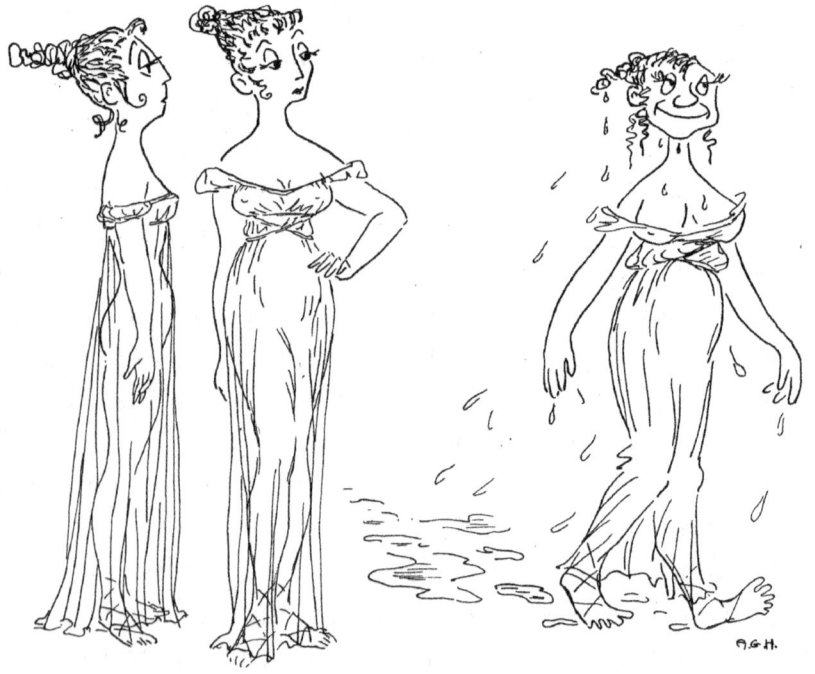

tive politicking in the streets and in the Forum. "Save the Mark!" This was for the repeal of the law. He winds up with a sour prophetic warning:

"Give rein to that headstrong creature, woman, that unbroken beast, and then hope that she herself will know where to stop her excesses! ... what they wish to have is freedom in all things or, rather, if we are to tell the truth, license in all things."

Spiro Agnew couldn't have said it any better.

So here we are in the {twenty-first} century still striving for freedom in all things. The Pill has liberated us from Victorian morals concerning sex, a mixed blessing from all accounts but the real freedom we need is from our own constricting misconceptions concerning our femaleness. As the archives prove, these mistaken beliefs are a tangled web of myths and old wives tales, some male-engendered, some not. We have been just as wrong in encouraging the earth-mother cult. The result is a sense of guilt if we don't or can't produce children.

This great stress put on productive wombs causes the worst mental anguish for us during menopause. Because bad habits are hard to change, we continue to brood like a flock of broody-hens. Oh to be a feckless spring-chicken again. Since that is not to be, let's swallow great doses of positive thinking and change the world along with ourselves.

CHAPTER TEN

This struggle of ours to rethink ourselves into the twenty-first century, scraping off the barnacles of inherited superstition as we go, is a very exciting one. Nothing like a clean bottom to make a vessel yar. While we are sailing around so nippily being pleased with ourselves, we can well afford to spare, some sympathy for our misused sisters of yore who suffered many more slings and arrows of outrageous fortune than we.

In the Seventh Century BC, Simonides wrote a scathing description of womankind, stating-that nine out of every ten women were worthless. Furthermore, they derived their nasty traits from animals. The uncleanly came from the sow, the exceedingly clever from the fox, the curious from the dog, the idle from the ass, the dull gourmand from the earth, the spiteful from the cat, the vain from the horse, the ugly from the apes and the capricious from the sea. The one and only good woman descended from the bee, who "loved and loving, grows old with her husband, the mother of a beautiful and famous race." (Of course, he knew nothing about bees.) Imagine trying to live down that propaganda for a few centuries.

Then we have a pithy tale by Herodotus in the Fourth Century BC. It seems that King Candanles was so proud of his wife's beauty that he wanted his best friend Gyges to see her naked. Gyges demurred so Candanles tricked him into viewing the beautiful Queen being undressed in her chambers. Her Majesty, struck dumb with shame momentarily, quickly gathered her wits and laid it on the line to Gyges:

"Either slay Candanles and become my lord and gain the kingdom of Lydia, or be content to die at once yourself where you are."

Gyges, no fool he, did as bid and gained a wife and kingdom on what otherwise might have been a very dull afternoon.

This may have been a first inkling of the Women's Liberation Movement but if people really do fashion their lives from the memory of the past, the experience of the present and the hope of the future, the ancient Greek women were up to their eyeballs in trouble. Even after marriage they had to fight for their husbands' attentions in competition with beautiful young men. Perhaps that is why they took to garments woven of Coan cloth, so transparent the wearer looked naked. In the Third Century BC Theocritus sniffily dubbed them as "wet garments." The popularity of this fabulous cloth from the Is-land of Cos was legendary. Rome's tart-tongued bisexual Seneca was still inveighing against it three centuries later. "Silken clothes, if they can be called clothes, which protect neither a woman's body nor her modesty ... so that our women may show as much of themselves to the world at large as they show to their lovers in the bedroom." One judges from this that the Roman matrons were busily having affairs in their diaphanous draperies.

Since Roman men seemed to prefer the company of the *hetairai*, (a good old Greek word: talented, well-educated women who believed in free love,) it is no wonder. Their wives also-faced the competition of young men as in Greece, though not to such an extent. Roman men, sensing which way the wind was blowing, passed a law that forbade aristocratic women to become prostitutes. Then to make sure everything was ship-shape they decreed that all prostitutes had to wear the toga (Man's dress) as their outer garment. The ladies of the evening were also forbidden to marry a senator or his descendant or a free-born man of Rome. On the other hand a procurer could become a Roman citizen; such was Roman justice. (The prostitutes who plied their trade in graveyards were called the *bustuarie*, who, when business was slow, hired themselves out as professional mourners — a nice change of pace.)

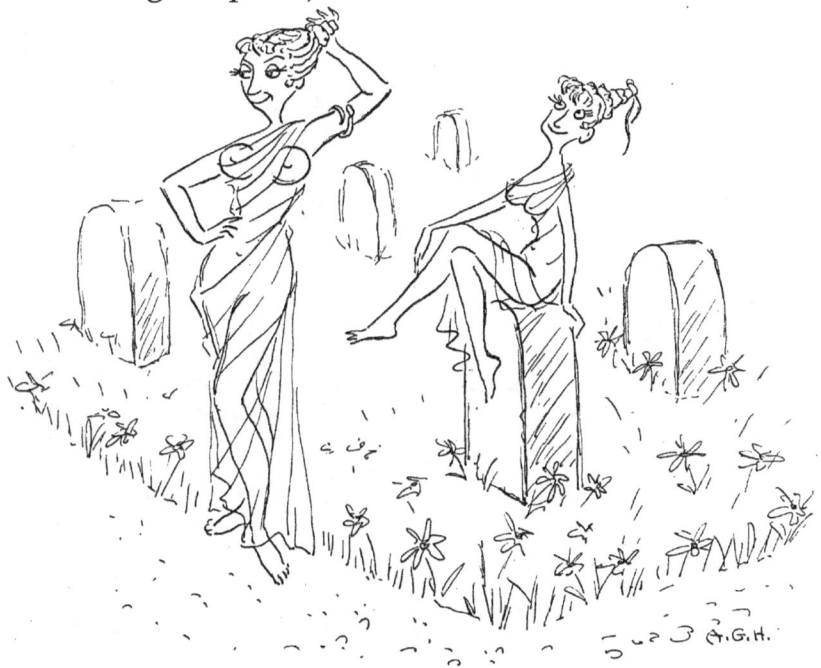

But Greek and Roman women were free as birds compared to the females of India four hundred years later.

In the Kama Sutra (circa 400 AD), Vatsyayana wrote endless rules of sexual behavior for both men and women. It makes The Sensuous Woman read like a nursery rhyme. In the case of men it was seduction all the way. In the case of women: compliance all the way, with grace. The rules for married women were very strict indeed. "As soon as she hears her lord's footsteps she should instantly leave whatever she is doing and rise, ready to obey his slightest desire. Then she must order her servants to wash his feet if she does not do so herself." The Kama Sutra continues with some rather sound counsel.

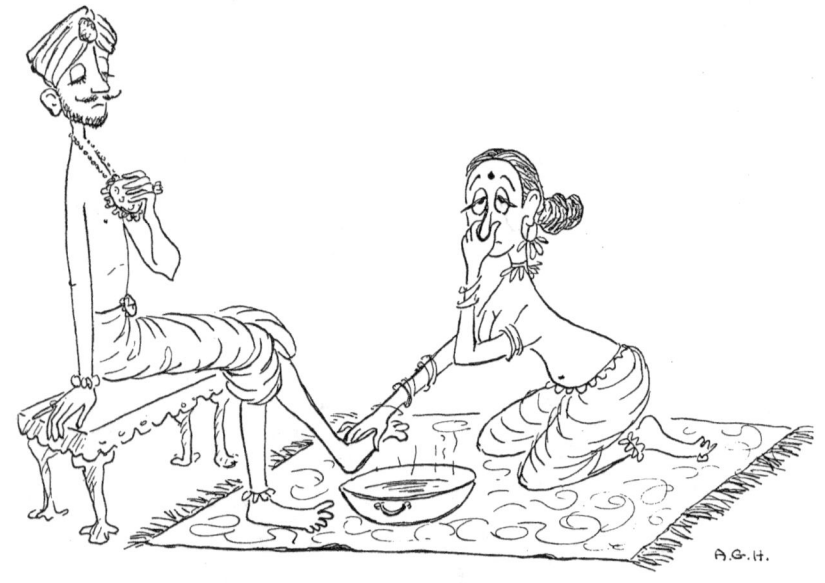

"When a wife desires union with her husband, she should dress herself in an ornate costume, put flowers in her hair, and wear vivid and exciting colors and perfume herself heavily with unguents and ointments."

A much harder piece of advice to accept was the admonition to the barren wife to recommend that her husband take a second spouse, give the newcomer a superior position in the household, and love her like a sister! This was only slightly offset by the fact that the second wife had to ask the first wife's permission to sleep with their mutual husband." What a tangled web that must have been.

It might have gotten tangled even further if the husband had used an aphrodisiac extolled by the Kama Sutra, to wit: "If a man rubs his *lingam* with a mixture of the powder of cactus, black pepper and honey, and then indulges in sexual intercourse, his partner will submit completely to his will and will never desire union with another."

Then there was "suttee"' (the concremation of a widow on her husband's funeral pyre) an old Indian custom. In the beginning it was a messy, mass immolation, as all the husband's wives, concubines, studs, etc., had to be burned together to maintain the dearly departed's status in the next world. What a way to go!

In fact, Indian women have had a thin time of it for millennia. Widows, no matter how young, were forbidden by Hindu custom to remarry or wear any jewelry, any cosmetics, any sari other than a plain white one, or to eat with the-family.

In ancient Peru females had an even worse time than in India. They were pawns owned by the government. If supplies of cloth were low, all the young females in one town might be transported to weaving nunneries to work from dawn to dusk. If concubines were needed instead, off they would be whisked in a different direction, to work from dusk to dawn. At least that was better than being chosen for human sacrifice, a custom that existed in all centuries someplace on our spinning world, from Greece to Mexico to

Polynesia to Africa. That was one problem we shared with men who were most welcome to their part of it.

Lots of problems were solely ours, however. If one were a member of the Trobriand tribe in northwestern Melanesia, and if one were caught in adultery, one would have to climb the tallest palm tree in sight and jump to one's just reward. The mind boggles at the thought of the splattered sidewalks that would decorate Palm Beach every day if such were the practice here.

On the plus side we have the special position accorded post-menopausal Balinese women until recently. The procreative years were considered dangerous and impure and women in this category were denied the right to take part in most ceremonies. After menopause however, these women were given special status, assisting in the ceremonies with the young virgins. They needed to be modest of speech and action no longer and were allowed to use obscene language more freely than any man. Maybe our young college dissidents are post-menopausal and don't know it.

The archives are crammed full of such lovely lore, telling us that we present-day females are very well off indeed. Every time we begin to doubt it we should grab a history book and start reading. We certainly would be provoked if our clitoris had been cut off to prevent our enjoying sex or if we had our vagina sewn up each time our husband left on a business trip, both of which used to happen in Africa.

One last juicy tidbit from ancient Rome. The Fescennine songs were sung by farmers while they carried a large carved phallus through the fields, the phallus being the symbol of nature's generative power. Fes-

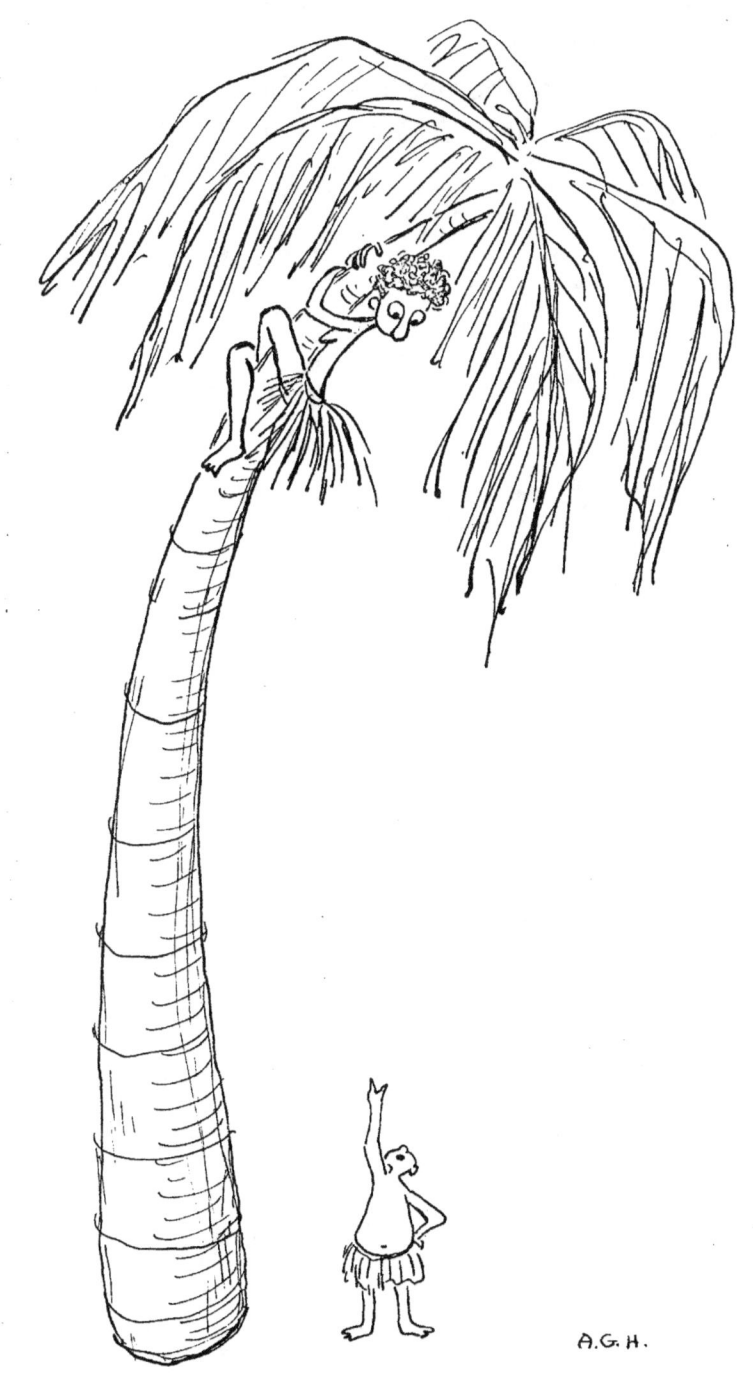

A.G.H.

cennine is derived from *fascinum*, one of the many names for phallus. Thus "fascinate" means "enchanted by the sight of the phallus." The whole thing fascinates me, so if that be penis envy, make the most of it.

CHAPTER ELEVEN

Cosmetics, women's best friend, have not always been in such good odor as they are now. In 1770 the English Parliament passed a law that said: "All women of whatever age, rank, profession or degree, whether virgins, maids or widows, that shall, from and after such act, dispose upon, seduce and betray into matrimony, any of His Majesty's subjects by the scents, paints, cosmetic washes, artificial teeth, false hair, Spanish wool, iron stays, hoops, high-heeled shoes, bolstered hips, shall incur the penalty of the law in force against witchcraft and like misdemeanors, and that the marriage, upon conviction, shall stand null and void."

Masculine liberation had reared its ugly head. The poor darlings must have been taken to the cleaners by droves before that.

English law notwithstanding, cosmetics had been, and continue to be, the non-caloric staff of life for any red-blooded female. We still do what our ancestresses did thousands of years ago: paint our faces, dye our hair, pluck our eyebrows — the whole schmear. If we were ancient Britons, we would probably even paint our bottoms blue like our husbands. A little sauce for the goose, and all that.

Now that we are facing menopause, cosmetics can serve a dual purpose in our lives improving both our physical and mental selves. Beauty aids have done their double duty since Eve snatched the original fig leaf.

The first record of cosmetics being used comes from Egypt 4,000 years ago. Toilet articles and unguents buried with the kings in their tombs attest to a lively interest in improving their appearance artificially. The Egyptians probably invented the bath as we know it, along with the perfumed oil massage that followed. Kohol was used extensively by the ladies to paint their eyes larger, being applied to lid, lashes and eyebrows. The underside of the eye was painted green. Henna was used to dye nails, palms of hands and feet, as is still done in parts of India today.

The derogatory term "Jezebel" all started "When Jehu was come to Jezreel, Jezebel heard of it; and she painted her face and tired her head and looked out at a window." (II Kings IX.30). Jezebel had made a tactical error, as she headed Jehu's pogrom list because of her raffish reputation. Jehu promptly told her two eunuchs to toss her out the window, which they did "and some of her blood was sprinkled on the wall, and on the horses: and he trode her under foot." Much later, after our hero "did eat and drink" he said, "Bury her: for she is a king's daughter." But by that time the only remnants left of the great beauty were her skull, feet, and the palms of her hands, all of which delighted Jehu who crowed, "This is the word of the Lord...in the portion of Jezreel shall dogs eat the flesh of Jezebels And the carcass of Jezebel shall be as dung upon the face of the field." All things considered, Jezebel should have kept her face clean, her mouth shut and her head away from the window.

By the time our old friends the Greeks and Romans had been fooling around with their phials full of philters for a few centuries, cosmetics as we know them today had practically arrived. White lead (which is still used in Europe, unfortunately,) and chalk whitened their skin. Egyptian Kohol darkened the eyelids and lashes, and fucus, a rouge, reddened cheeks and lips. Psilotrum was a species of depilatory, barley flour and butter cured blemishes and pumice stone brightened the teeth. They bleached their hair with a soap imported from Gaul. The dark-haired ladies had gone mad for blond and red tresses the minute they saw the first fair-haired slave from the north.

So it went, with questionable improvements through the centuries, until the great scientific breakthrough of our time. We are lucky indeed to have the Food and Drug Administration (FDA), a beady-eyed protector who checks the ingredients put in our cosmetics with fanatical zeal. The Elizabethan lip rouge made from red crystalline mercuric sulphide would never pass muster now. It was very effective, as long as you had any lips left on which to pit it. Mercuric sulphide has an unhappy tendency to eat away flesh.

The FDA would be just as leery of burned jawbone of hog, flowers of brimstone, distilled raven, oil of turpentine, sublimate of mercury, powdered brick and coral used on skin and teeth, or calcined lead, sulphur and quick lime mixed for a hair bleach. How about a brilliantine made from apple pressings left over from cider-making mixed with hog's grease? The Madison Avenue boys would really tear up their head rugs on that one. No wonder when Queen Elizabeth I died she left "80 wigs of divers colours."

But our guardian dragon, the FDA, makes sure that we will never suffer from any sublimate of mercury poisoning or eye of newt allergy, bless their hearts.

The American Medical Association is another anchor to windward in the stormy waters of the drug

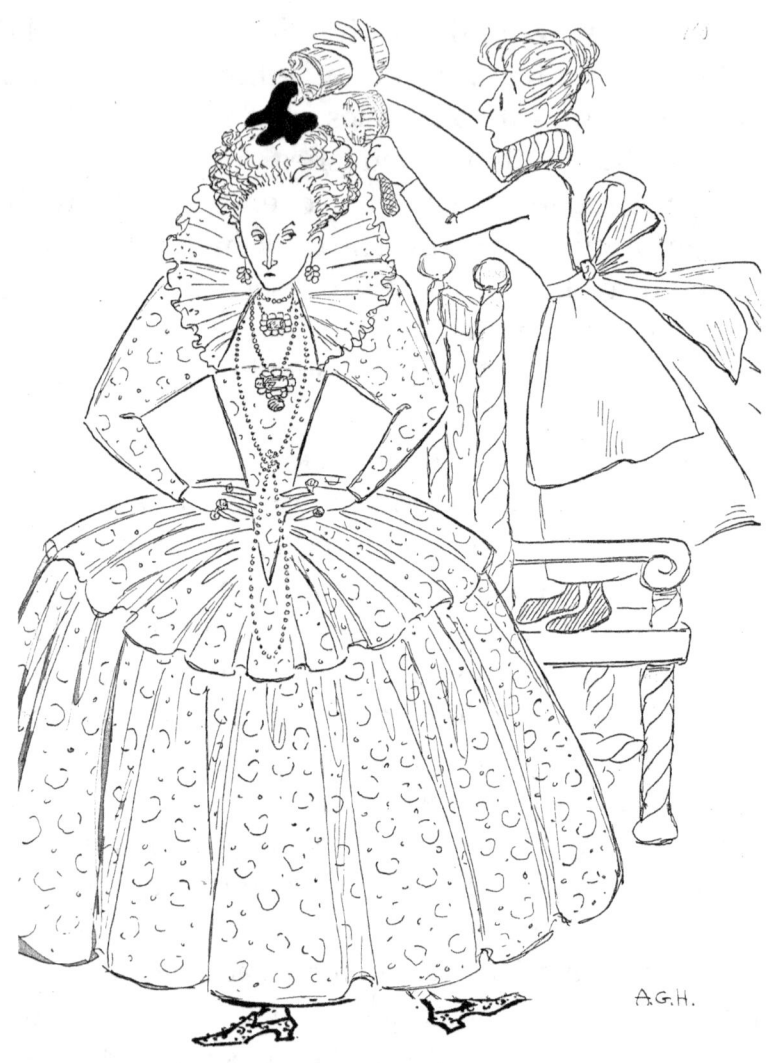

business. The organization's magazine, Today's Health, tells females exactly what they can and cannot expect cosmetics and surgery to do for them, among other things. Doctors readily agree that there are ways "to retard or lessen unwanted changes in your skin," i.e., wrinkles and roughness, but there is no way to stop the aging process. There is no miracle cream that will safely and effectively remove wrinkles, flowery promises to the contrary. But there are several things we can do to minimize and delay our wrinkles as long as possible.

The first and foremost of these, which all doctors stress heavily, is to avoid excessive exposure to the sun. Dermatologists believe that old-looking skin may be due more to the effects of the sun than to the aging process itself. Ultra-violet rays cause chronic and irreversible degenerative changes in the skin, especially in persons with fair complexions, who have less melanin (pigment) in their skin to protect them. So either stay out of the sun entirely or use a tanning lotion with a sun screening ingredient, constantly and lavishly. Don't bake for hours in the sun, either. You'll not only save yourself a wrinkled weather-beaten face but you may also save yourself skin cancer. Sunlight is a major factor in causing that disease. Victorian ladies with their summer mittens and parasols were on the side of the angels. The second most important thing to do is use face creams or lotions containing emollients for softening and soothing, and humectants for attracting and retaining moisture. Those are the vital ingredients. The medical profession doesn't seem to put much stock in face creams containing hormones, royal jelly or turtle oil, et al, doing any extra magic, as it can't be scientifically proved that they are better. It can't be definitely disproved either, so if you have a favorite hormone, or whatever cream that you like, use it. It intrigues me that doctors will deny the efficacy of hormone creams on the face, and yet prescribe hormone creams to build up and soften the vagina walls if they become thinner after menopause. Oh well. To each his own mystique.

The third thing to remember is that all the creams in the world, hormonal or not, won't do you any good whatsoever, unless they are used regularly and without fail. If you started using face cream in your twenties you were a smart girl, indeed. Even smarter if you combined it with nightly neck exercises. Half your problem is solved already,

If you like massage, face masks and facial isometric exercises, go right ahead. There doesn't seem to be proof positive that they help, but they don't do any harm. If they make you feel better, well that's the idea behind all cosmetics. Besides, something must work, as we all know women in their fifties or sixties who look twenty years younger.

It is this desire to feel and look our best that has made plastic surgery such a psychological boon to humankind. Dumbo-ears, turkey-gobbler necks, baggy eyes, sagging faces, saddle-seat rear ends can all be improved by a clever scalpel. Plastic surgery has an old and honorable history going back to ancient Egypt and India. Doctors feel it was probably the very first form of surgery known to man, and man dreamed up sane dillies to improve himself.

In the Kama Sutra, for instance, it says that if a man feels that his sexual prowess needs a shot in the arm, so to speak, he can pierce a hole in the end of his penis, sit in water until the bleeding has stopped, and then indulge in very active intercourse so that the hole can be cleansed. (The whole A.M.A. has just fainted.) When the hole has healed, any amount of interesting objects can be inserted to make the act of love a really ticklish affair. Other Asian men discovered that by making a circle of slits instead of just one, plac-
92

ing pebbles inside and allowing the skin to heal over them, they had a formidable tool to conjure with. The Burmese went one step further and added bells instead of stones. "Keeping time, time, time; in a sort of Runic rhyme, to the tintinnabulation that so musically wells, from the bells, bells, bells, bells, bells, bells, bells; from the jingling and the tingling of the bells."

Doe-eyed Indian women contented themselves with merely slitting the outer edges of babies girls' eyes to make them appear larger. This was the reverse of the women of New Guinea who shaved off their eyebrows and bit off each others' eyelashes to make their eyes look small; a sign of great beauty.

Skimpy eyes or saucer eyes make no difference today. The tiniest orbs can be made to sparkle plenty with modern make-up, so the plastic surgeon is saved at least one operation. What he does do with his expertise is put many a bitter, unhappy person back in circulation again, feeling and looking like a new woman or man, as the case may be. In Sweden you

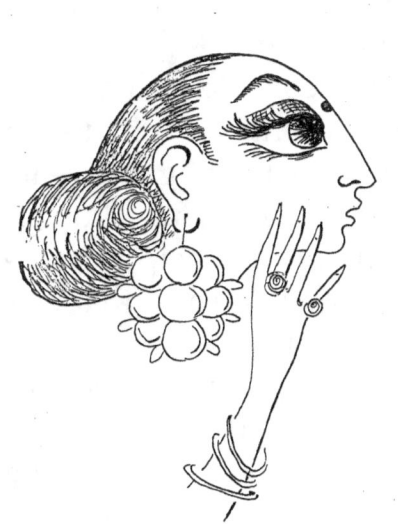
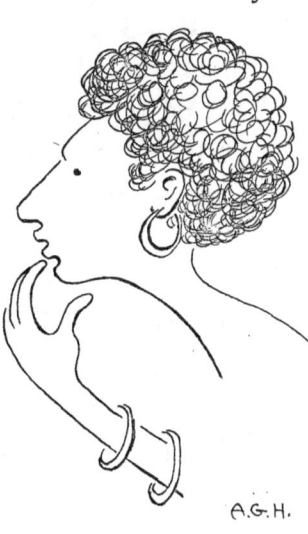

A.G.H.

can have the best of both worlds. If it becomes absolutely vital to one's well-being, any hesitation about going under the knife is ridiculous. The A.M.A. has published a guide to the general price of some of the most popular operations.

Nose: $500 to $1,000, face lift: $750 to $3,000, eyelids: $400 to $750, ears: $350 to $600, breasts (reduction): $750 to $1,500, breasts (augmentation): $500 to $750. {As of 1973.} I'm sure that it would be more than $1,500 to fix the bosoms of certain African women who have had their breasts elongated from puberty so that they can easily feed babies slung on their backs.

Even before one trots into the operating room, figuratively speaking, one can improve a bad skin by both dermabrasion, a sandpaper-like technique for removing the top-most layer of skin or Chemabrasion, the same thing done with chemicals. Both these procedures must be performed by experts, as they have to be done with the utmost care. Also, unwanted hair can be removed by electrolysis or a depilatory. Otherwise, trim your whiskers with manicure scissors, don't pluck them, as tweezing can start skin infections.

Lots of woman would never consider plastic surgery for themselves; at least not until they had seen their best friend suddenly appear looking ten years younger. Again, it is all a matter of our psychological makeup. What we actually need is help to make us feel like complete, well rounded persons (that was not meant as a pun, but let it go.) We don't have to feel guilty if we either want, or don't want, a younger face and body than nature has decreed. Every life is a very complex voyage into the unknown, and we have to choose our own individual ways to cope with it.

94

With or without the reassurance of a mirror, if we know ourselves to be vital and attractive, we can face big bags full of wildcats — they won't have a chance.

CHAPTER TWELVE

According to anthropologist Margaret Meade, all we females, with a few eccentric exceptions, are born absolutely sure of our femininity. We find out early on that we are like our mothers, we girls: no doubt about it. It is a state of being. Our virginity is an irrefutable fact until some eager male proves it by disproving it. Our wombs carry babies: another absolute. All of this is accepted by us and those around us.

On the other hand the poor male finds out early in life that he is not like his mother — the most important person in his life. He then is faced with endless steps to be taken to become like his father: boys don't cry, boys are athletic, boys must dominate, etc. Males

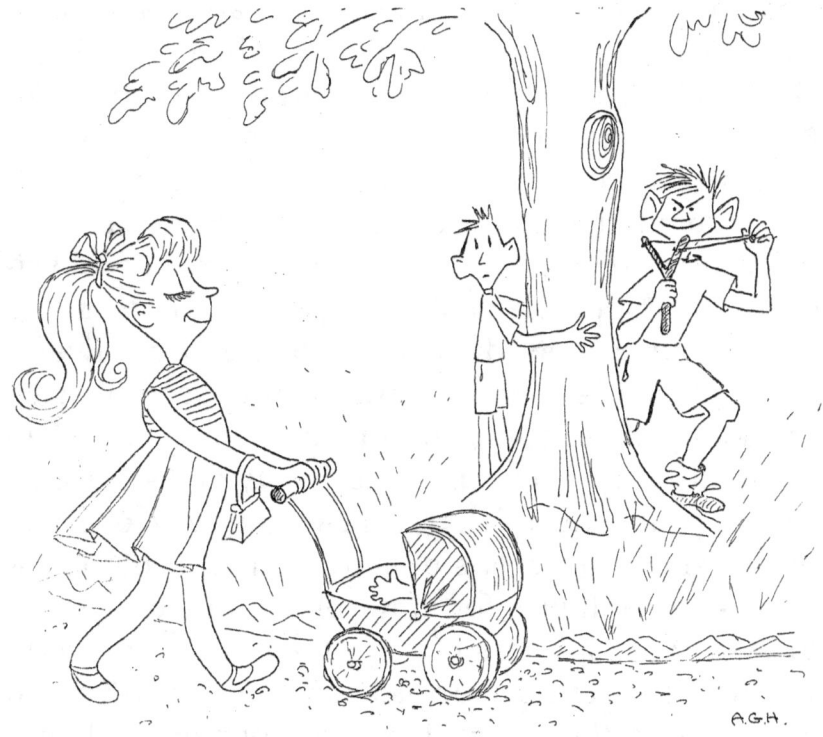

A.G.H.

eventually have to know a female sexually to attain their manhood. Even becoming a father is a dubious test, as no man can actually prove that he is the father, whereas the personal fact of motherhood is quite obvious to all concerned. {Today there are blood tests for DNA.} We *are*, and men have to *become*, which is all of a piece with Bucky Fuller's theory. This serene assurance of ours may be irritating to the opposite sex, but it is the rock upon which we build our personalities.

Dr. Meade also points out that one of "the particular characteristics of a changing society is the possibility of a deferred maturity, of later and later shifts in the lives of the most complex, the most flexible individuals."

In other words, we can still grow, regardless of age. I had a mother who became a dietician at age forty-nine and I have an aunt who taught herself both ancient and modern Greek in her fifties, so I knew Dr. Meade's theory to be a fact. It cheers me up no end. This inbuilt ability of ours to learn and change will never be put to better use than during menopause.

Evan for the 80% of women who have no physical or mental problems it is as good a time as any to stretch out in new directions. Dr. Reuben's Everything...About Sex points out that lack of use will make sexual organs atrophy, and the same thing applies to the brain. It will get dusty and musty and stale. One should really furnish one's head the way one furnishes one's house: lots of sturdy basic furniture for ease, some antiques for atmosphere, modern covers to wear well, splashes of color for gaiety and everywhere special bric-a-brac picked up on our travels, to add spice to the whole. However, our brain should be like Hadrian's villa, too: an endless series of rooms added on until the day we die. We won't have Hadrian's construction bills to pay, either.

For those who yearn for the Halls of Academe, go back and get your M.A. or PhD. Why not? If your husband or children object, sling a little Women's Lib lingo and watch them wilt. That poor old skinned cat is about to lose his shirt again.

You can also learn by doing as well as by studying. That's where sweet charity comes in. You have the added satisfaction of having another star in your crown when you get to heaven. Not to be sneezed at.

It used to be that we died about the same time our ovaries did, thrifty Mother Mature leaving no clutter. Now modern science has given us a bonus of a good thirty years more. It behooves us to see that this gift is an asset, not a liability.

While we are busy scampering over this watershed in our lives, let's not forget our families, poor darlings. All this preoccupation with our interiors can become quite a burden for those around us to share as we become increasingly egocentric. You will get a lot more sympathy if you explain just what is going on and why, especially to the man in your life. Men are basically very sympathetic creatures, if they think it is deserved. What they hate are surprises.

A weeping wife at the comedy of the season, at scalper's prices, will enrage any husband. A sudden temper tantrum just as he is taking his first bits of tenderloin will accomplish the same thing. Tired and hungry after a rough day at work, a man wants peace and quiet and a stiff drink. That's what he wants. What he gets is anyone's guess if a sudden spurt of estrogen has just entered his wife's bloodstream. If he knows that some days you will probably actively dislike him for no known reason, at least he can prepare his line of retreat to the den. When he starts to complain of mistreatment, quote a couplet written by Catullus. Catullus wrote it to an unfaithful mistress, but no matter: the sentiment is perfect.

"I hate and love. You ask how that can be?

I know not, but I feel the agony."

You may just get another muttered "Bull Manure" but at least you've given him pause. To return to our shattered husbands — poor lambs — women truly are difficult to live with, and when we are upset we're impossible. As long as we know it, they know it, and they know that we know they know it, the ground rules can be worked out. Why pull the tail of a maddened lion?

We have learned to avoid a simmering mate through sad experience. So can they. For our part, we can also exert some self control, as hard as that may be. In fact, most frustrating if you're just spoiling for a good fight, but never mind. A man may have lots of sympathy, but he doesn't have much patience. You'll have to find that fine line between.

The most important tiling to remember is to cheer yourself up in whatever way works best for you. Bath oils, perfumes, chic sunglasses, a new pants suit or whatever can all work minor miracles in this department. Try it and see. I love to spray cologne on my hair in the morning before I pin up my French twist, so that at night when I take it down I'm surrounded by a cloud of fragrance. If external trappings leave you cold, then feed the inner woman with studies of a new subject. One need not preclude the other. A face lift or a Ph.D are only two of myriad ways to assure and insure our individuality.

We females are much greater than the sum of our parts, as Bucky Fuller would be the first to admit. Furthermore, he would have a complete theoretical equation to back up the statement. But we know it intuitively. Chop out a uterus, trim off a double chin, paste on false eyelashes, snap on a padded bra, put some initials after our name…who cares? We are us. Invincible. Unique. That is why we have been beguiling the opposite sex since the beginning of time. That is why we will continue to do so. After all, Fe means iron in chemistry, a most durable substance.

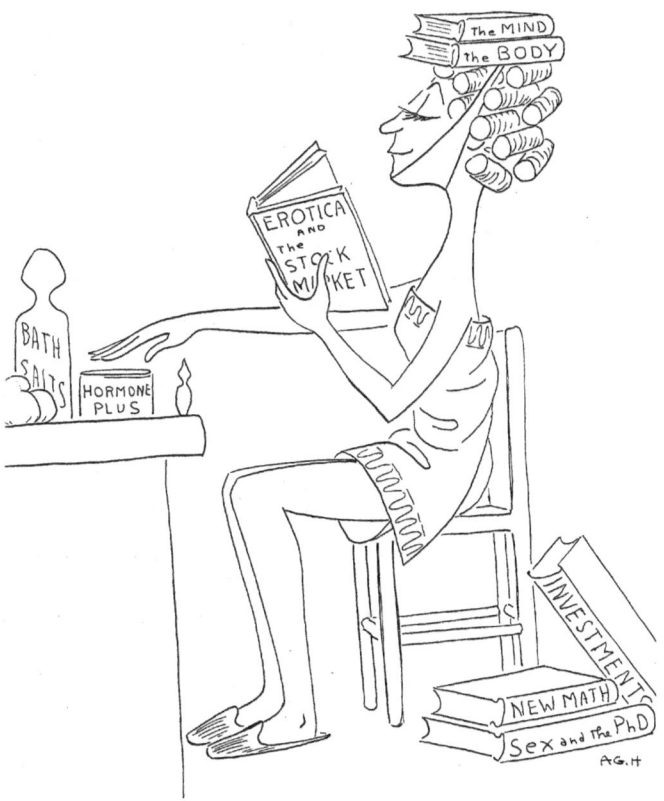

Therefore, be not of faint heart, my darlings: menopause is a temporary situation, thank God. Keep your sense of humor above all else. And while laughing with tears streaming down your face, you can say bravely, "Menopause can be fun!"

Bibliography for
Menopause Can Be Fun.
By Allene G. Hatch

1. *The Psychology of Women* by Helen Deutch, M.D. Grune & Stratton, 1945.

2. *Medical Psychology* by Gregory Zilboarg. W.W. Norton & Co., 1941.

3. *Textbook of Gynecology* by John I. Brewer. C.V. Mosbyio; St. Louis. 1966.

4. *The Textbook of Medical Physiology* by Arthur C. Guyton, M.D., W.B. Saunders Co., Philadelphia & London. 1966.

5. *The Hormone Quest* by Albert Q. Maisel. Random House. New York. 1965.

6. *Gynecologic Endocrinology* by Gardner M. Riley, Ph.D. A. Hoeber. Harper Books. 1959

7. *Gynecology and Gynecologic Nursing* by Miller and Avery. W.B. Saunders Co., Philadelphia & London. 1965.

8. *Principles of Obstetrics and Gynecology for Nurses* by Josephine Iorio. C.V. Mosby Co., St. Louis. 1967.

9. *Gynecologic Nursing* Brewer, Mollo and Gerlie. C.V. Mosby Co., St. Louis. 1966.

10. *Woman* by Dr. Joyce Brothers. Doubleday & Co., New York. 1961.

11. *Modern Woman's Medical Encyclopedia* edited by Anna Mantel Fishbein. Doubleday & Co., New York. 1966.

12. *The Sexual Life of Savages in North Western Melanesia* by Bronislaw Malinowski. Harcourt, Brace & World. 1929

13. *Sex Habits of The American Male* by Albert Deutsch. Prentice Hall. New York. 1948.

14. *Sexual Behavior in The Human Male* by Alfred Charles Kinsey, Wardell B. Pomeroy and Clyde E. Martin. W. B. Saunders Co., Philadelphia. 1948.

15. *Successful Marriage* by Morris Fishbein and Ernest W. Burgess. Doubleday & Co., Garden City. 1947.

16. *Kama Sutra of Vatsyayana*, Lancer Books, Inc. New York. 1964,

17. *Sexual Life in Ancient Greece* by Hans Licht. George Routledge & Sons, Ltd. London. 1932.

18. *Sexual Life in Ancient Rome* by Otto Kiefer. Barnes & Noble. New York. 1056

19. *Sex and Temperament in Three Primitive Societies* by Margaret Mead. New American Library. New York. 1963.

20. *Male and Female* by Margaret Mead. W. Marrow. New York. 1949.

21. *Everything You Always Wanted to Know About Sex* by David Reuben, M.D. David McKay Co., Inc. New York. 1970.

22. *Any Woman Can* by David Reuben, M.D. David McKay Co., Inc. New York. 1971

23. *The Pageant of Elizabethan England* by Elizabeth Burton. Charles Scribner's Sons. 1958.

24. *In Defense of Women* by H. L. Menken. A.A. Knopf. New York. 1924.

25. *Daughter to Napoleon* by Constance Wright. Holt, Rinehart & Winston. New York. 1961

26. *Search The Scriptures* by Robert B. Greenblatt, M.D. J. B. Lippincott Co. Philadelphia & Montreal. 1963.

27. *The Feminine Mystique* by Betty Friedan. W.W. Norton & Co., Inc. New York. 1963.

28. *The Female Eunuch* by Germaine Greer. McGraw-Hill Book Co., New York. 1971

29. *The Mature Woman* by Anna Kleegman Daniels, M.D. Prentice-Hall. New York.1953.
30. *Intimate Behavior* by Desmond Morris. Random House. New York. 1971

Articles by Buckminster Fuller; also interviews with Buckminster Fuller, Dr. David Block, Dr. Frank Smith, Dr. Desmond Heath, Dr. A. LaMarr Matthews and Dr. Thomas Young.

As of 2010 this book was checked for accuracy by Dr. Harlan Root.